SIDE EFFECTS

SIDE EFFECTS

How Our Healthcare Lost its Way – And How We Can Fix it

DAVID HASLAM

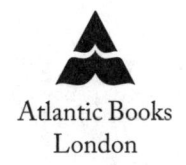

Atlantic Books
London

First published in hardback in Great Britain in 2022 by Atlantic Books, an imprint of Atlantic Books Ltd.

Copyright © David Haslam, 2022

The moral right of David Haslam to be identified as the author of this work has been asserted by him in accordance with the Copyright, Designs and Patents Act of 1988.

All rights reserved. No part of this publication may be reproduced, stored in a retrieval system, or transmitted in any form or by any means, electronic, mechanical, photocopying, recording, or otherwise, without the prior permission of both the copyright owner and the above publisher of this book.

1 2 3 4 5 6 7 8 9

A CIP catalogue record for this book is available from the British Library.

Hardback ISBN: 978-1-78649-536-5
E-Book ISBN: 978-1-78649-538-9
Paperback ISBN: 978-1-78649-539-6

Printed in Great Britain by Bell and Bain Ltd, Glasgow

Atlantic Books
An imprint of Atlantic Books Ltd
Ormond House
26–27 Boswell Street
London
WC1N 3JZ

www.atlantic-books.co.uk

For my family

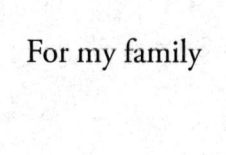

Contents

Foreword — 1

Chapter 1: We've Got a Problem — 9

Chapter 2: How Did We Get Here? — 38

Chapter 3: Paying the Price — 64

Chapter 4: Why Is it All So Expensive? — 84

Chapter 5: Valuing a Life — 110

Chapter 6: Better than Cure — 134

Chapter 7: Overtreatment and Overdiagnosis — 155

Chapter 8: Hearts and Minds — 180

Chapter 9: Age and Ageing — 190

Chapter 10: And in the End … — 206

Chapter 11: Care in the Future — 217

Chapter 12: A Way Forward — 238

Acknowledgements — 261
Endnotes — 262
Index — 287

Foreword

I've spent my life working in healthcare. For many years, I was involved in both devising and implementing many aspects of local and national health policy, and I've also experienced it first-hand, as a patient. From every perspective, there is clearly a mismatch between supply and demand. While resources can never be infinite, the demand for healthcare in Britain appears to be inexhaustible. This imbalance is a source of immense tension, and the situation is only getting worse. In this book, I will first assess this extraordinary challenge and then attempt to suggest how we might tackle it.

In the past few years, the NHS has faced a double whammy; first the government's pursuit of austerity reduced its capacity and then the immense challenge of Covid-19 tested it to its limits. Even before this, it faced massive and unsustainable pressure. While increased funding is critically important, it cannot be the only solution to every problem.

The coronavirus pandemic has, to an unprecedented degree, devastatingly exposed the challenge that is facing us. For a while, it trumped everything else, and not just in Britain. All around the world, governments recognized the supreme importance of health and healthcare, as well as the key role that the state has to play in protecting its citizens.

In ancient Rome, the statesman Cicero wrote that 'the health of the people is the supreme law'. Two thousand years later, as the UK stood on the brink of crisis in March 2020, the Chancellor of the Exchequer Rishi Sunak said, 'Whatever extra resources our NHS needs to cope with Covid-19, it will get. Whatever it needs, whatever it costs, we stand behind our NHS.' In countries around the world, politicians displayed the same sentiment. Funds somehow appeared, and no expense was spared. Repeated comparisons were made to the challenges of wartime. In March 2020, the prime minister Boris Johnson declared that his government would act 'like any other wartime governments' to support the British economy and take 'steps that are unprecedented since World War II'.[1] Other world leaders used similar descriptions. The US president Donald Trump referred to himself as a 'wartime president' and Andrew Cuomo, governor of New York, reportedly said that 'ventilators are to this war what bombs were to World War II'.[2]

The battle with disease – with a single disease that spread easily and posed a particular threat to the eldest and most vulnerable – was in full swing. Humankind had to fight this virus with whatever weapons it could muster, which initially meant prioritizing healthcare over the needs of the economy and all the other various priorities that usually jostle for attention. It was extraordinary, but it was necessary. However, things were far from typical. Funds are not infinite, and they never can be. In more normal times, when we are not facing a global pandemic, we still find ourselves having to make life-and-death choices. After all, healthcare can be massively expensive. Every year, the cost of care escalates, and the money has to be found to pay for it. Even prior to the pandemic, in 2017, the UK spent £197 billion on healthcare, equating to £2,989 per person.[3] Research scientists continue to develop new drugs and therapies;

the potential benefits that they offer to humankind are phenomenal, but the accompanying prices almost inevitably go up and up.

Even before Covid-19, the proportion of national wealth that was spent on healthcare was increasing every year, and every prediction of future trends showed that this challenge was only going to worsen. Although this issue is facing every country on earth, we seem remarkably reluctant to discuss it. Society might in the short term have debates about whether a particular amount of spending is sufficient, but we rarely consider the longer-term perspective. Burying our heads in the sand and ignoring a deepening problem can never be a sensible long-term policy, however tempting it might be.

However, the increasing cost of care isn't our only challenge. Of the diseases that posed the greatest threat to the average family just a few decades ago, many have now been eradicated. Life expectancy has also increased since then, yet people are as anxious about their health as ever, and there has been no let-up in demand for the medical profession, particularly for reassurance. A hundred and fifty years ago, a typical day's work for a British general practitioner would have consisted of a constant stream of patients with pneumonia (which was frequently fatal), diphtheria, cholera and acute rheumatism, in addition to the flood of minor problems that all family doctors would still recognize today.[4] Today's GPs might look at that workload from a previous age and notice that almost all these illnesses have either been wiped out or are now eminently treatable. They might find themselves wondering what would be left for them to do, but as some challenges have been eliminated, new problems have arisen to take their place. Family doctors today are busier than they have ever been – and this is discounting the impact of the Covid pandemic. So, what is going on? Can we foresee a world where healthcare facilities sit unused while a healthy and happy population has no need for care? Or will the predictions that envisage perpetually rising expectations and demand prove to be accurate? If they do, is this a sustainable model? And what is driving it?

This dilemma is the subject of this book. If we can accept that there will never be enough money to cover every possible eventuality – and it's hard to imagine that there ever could be – how should society make choices? What is the real value of healthcare, and what is the endgame? Disease and infirmity will never disappear completely, so we need to ask ourselves whether we are using the available funds in the best possible way. When can it be justifiable to spend more money on healthcare, if that means taking money away from other areas of our lives, which might include education or even security? This was another challenge that was thrown into sharp focus by Covid. When populations were locked down, although they were relatively safe from direct impact by the virus, the restrictions had a damaging impact on happiness, education, physical health, mental health and wellbeing. Governments found themselves having to balance the dangers of the virus with the dangers of lockdown. If a country's economy suffers, a major impact on its population's health will follow. And conversely, if the health of the nation suffers, there will be a major negative impact on the economy. So how can we decide where our priorities should lie?

The problem is a global one, and in the long term, simply increasing healthcare spending is unlikely to be the sole solution. That said, the challenges facing the National Health Service in the UK have been exacerbated by a decade or more of underfunding; I should emphasize that I will most definitely *not* argue in this book that British healthcare currently has enough money. Years of austerity following the global financial crisis of 2008 have had a major impact. Waiting lists had risen to 4.6 million even before

Covid attacked, and staffing levels were clearly becoming seriously inadequate.[5] As the wide-ranging LSE–Lancet Commission on the future of the NHS made very clear, the Covid-19 pandemic has reinforced the economic case for investing in health, which is crucial for both fiscal sustainability and societal wellbeing.[6] The commission estimated that in order to implement its funding recommendations, total expenditure on the NHS would need to increase by around £102 billion in real terms, which will represent around 3.1 per cent of the UK's gross domestic product in 2030–31.

In September 2021, Boris Johnson announced a new funding settlement for health and social care in England, which included an additional £6.6 billion for NHS England in 2022–23 and £3.6 billion in 2023–24 – on top of the plans made before the pandemic – as a result of ongoing pressures from Covid-19. Few people working in healthcare felt that this would be sufficient. Even the Institute for Fiscal Studies stated that while the extra funding would help for about two years, it was unlikely to be sufficient in the medium term.[7]

These are eye-watering sums, and there is no doubt that the NHS is facing an uphill struggle if it is to catch up once the pandemic is over. But it is equally clear that in the longer term, a more fundamental reconsideration of how we perceive healthcare is required. Indeed, while the population has, in general, never been healthier, we seem to consider ourselves to be more at risk of falling ill than ever – and we are more anxious about our health than at any time in our history. Despite all the advances we are making in our ability to diagnose and treat illness, the demand on healthcare services continues to rise inexorably.

The key question I will return to throughout this book is a simple one. What is it that we are really trying to achieve through our healthcare system? And if we have a goal in mind, are we going the right way about trying to achieve it?

Today, many aspects of human existence are at risk of being medicalized – another side effect of the hard-won successes of modern medicine. But is this really healthy? Is it logical? And is it beneficial? In the future, it may be that we look back on current events and realize that the pandemic opened our eyes to this challenge. With the vast level of government spending that Covid-19 triggered, having threatened the long-term sustainability of health systems, we need to find ways of doing more with less. We have an opportunity to ensure we are focused on doing the right things, and we should as a priority tackle overmedicalization and the unnecessary tests, diagnoses and therapies that can potentially cause harm as well as leading to waste – not just of money, but of time and expertise.

Again, I must stress that this is absolutely *not* a book about how we should fund our healthcare systems in the short term. In most countries, the pandemic has caused immense urgent challenges, whether because of the potential impact of long Covid, the huge disruption that it has caused to other aspects of care or its massive impact on a nation's economy. However, in the medium to long term, it is vital that we look at how healthcare is evolving and try to define the role it should play in a modern society. What is it that we are really trying to achieve?

It is clear that many of the determinants of health, far from having anything to do with healthcare, are profoundly linked to social factors such as education or poverty. When does society decide that problems require healthcare input, and when should they be treated as societal issues? We could continue to spend ever-increasing sums, but it must be clear what we are hoping to achieve. While I am absolutely not a health economist, I have observed these challenges first-hand and from all manner of perspectives.

If you have infinite wealth or live in a country with an unlimited healthcare budget, then these questions won't apply to you. But my guess is that you don't. Healthcare costs are perpetually escalating all over the world, and these are real challenges that will affect the vast majority of people on the planet. And this isn't a book about what some people have called 'death panels', about how governments might callously determine who deserves to be treated and who will be left to die. It's not about rationing – it's about rationality. It's not about theoretical fears – it's about a real world that we need to face up to – and now.

This is a vital debate, and it won't go away with wishful thinking. My hope is that this book will ask important questions and begin to suggest some answers.

David Haslam
April 2022

CHAPTER 1

We've Got a Problem

In late March 2020, the planet seemed on the brink of catastrophe, as the Covid-19 pandemic threatened to overwhelm health services around the world. In the UK, inspired by the speed with which the Chinese government had designed and built a 1,000-bed hospital in Wuhan, the city where the virus first emerged, a group of military planners and staff from NHS England visited ExCeL Exhibition Centre in east London's Docklands. Just three days later, on 24 March, the health secretary Matt Hancock announced plans to convert the conference centre into a 4,000-bed unit, the first in a series of what were to be called 'Nightingale hospitals'.[1] The scale and speed of the development was breathtaking; on 3 April, Prince Charles formally opened the impressive new facility via video link. As a demonstration of determined action in the face of a terrifying pandemic, it was just what the nation needed.

However, after the initial drama, and a raft of enthusiastic headlines, none of these facilities solved the problems they had been designed for. Of the seven Nightingale hospitals that were built in England, only three ever actually treated patients; by January 2021, these hospitals had between them treated a total of 272 patients, despite a cost to the taxpayer of more than £500 million. The facilities in Birmingham, Sunderland, Bristol and Harrogate didn't treat a single Covid-19 inpatient during that time.[2] London's

Nightingale hospital was closed in May 2020, having treated just fifty-one patients, although it was subsequently repurposed in January 2021 to take patients without Covid-19, in order to relieve the pressure on beds in the capital's other hospitals.

The reason for the facilities' apparent failure was straightforward: the UK simply didn't have the trained nursing staff and other personnel to work in them. Delivering healthcare always needs people, and in spring 2020 the people just weren't there. Years of damaging austerity, combined with a serious pre-existing workforce crisis, had left the NHS with precious little spare capacity when it came to staff. While the achievement of designing and building the Nightingales in a matter of days was truly impressive, without enough doctors, nurses, personal protective equipment, ventilators and respiratory therapists to work in them, it was a gesture that was as empty as the hospitals would prove to be.

The long-term challenge
I do not intend to use hindsight to criticize the many difficult and urgent decisions that were made in the midst of a crisis. Nor is this a book about how healthcare systems should attempt to recover from the impact of the pandemic, about how we should tackle the challenge of social care and the backlog of non-Covid cases that the former NHS chief executive Sir David Nicholson has described as 'truly frightening'. These are clearly all incredibly important issues, but behind them lie a number of even more thought-provoking long-term questions.

My aim is to examine the long-term challenges that are facing every healthcare system in the world. While the pandemic has opened our eyes to the magnificent achievements of modern science, it has also focused attention on the challenges that we face when demand for healthcare outstrips supply. In the early days of the pandemic, the world watched in horror at what was happening in northern Italy, where doctors found themselves having to make life-and-death decisions based on the availability of beds and staff. When we don't have the necessary resources to provide all the care that people might need, what do we do? And what *should* we do?

After all, this isn't a problem that will only arise during a pandemic. The cost of healthcare is escalating almost everywhere in the world, as is the demand for care. Thanks to advances in science, both the offers and the expectations of what can be achieved are growing, but however much we may wish it were otherwise, there will never be enough money to pay for everything. A World Health Organization report concluded that healthcare spending is growing faster than the economy in nearly every country it looked at.[3] So how do we make the right choices when it comes to healthcare spending? What gives us the best bang for our buck?

Covid-19 has dramatically heightened our awareness of the social determinants of health, and in particular the damaging impact of deprivation. In the UK, black, Asian and minority ethnic groups were far more likely to die in the pandemic than the white majority. And according to the Office for National Statistics, the Covid mortality rate in the most deprived places in England was double that of the least deprived areas. A report by the All Party Parliamentary Group on Longevity titled 'Levelling Up Health' and published in April 2021 warned that the UK has the 'worst population health in Europe', and concluded that this was partly responsible for the tragically high number of Covid-19 deaths.[4] If mortality rates in all local areas of England had been as low as in the least deprived localities, the number of deaths would have been 35 per cent lower. Deprivation kills, and it was clear that we hadn't all been in it together.

The same pattern was repeated all around the world. In the US, research showed that residents of the most disadvantaged counties were at a dramatically increased risk of death.[5] In Spain, data published by the Catalonian government suggested that the rate of Covid-19 infection was six or seven times higher in the most deprived areas of the region than in the least deprived.[6] Likewise in Brazil, the burden of Covid-19 has been greater in areas with high social deprivation.[7] And in Sweden, studies have shown that being male, having less disposable income, a lower level of education, not being married and having immigrated from a low- or middle-income country all independently predict a higher risk of death from Covid-19.[8]

It should be obvious by now that the solution to this immense challenge is not simply to build more hospitals, which may make for good headlines but doesn't necessarily solve the problems. It is also critical that healthcare systems have the capacity to face future emergencies, even if we don't know what they are. Early in my career as a doctor, I learned that the one thing that you could predict with certainty was that something unpredictable would happen almost daily. As a result, it was vital to build in both the time and the capacity to deal with unforeseen events – running everything at full capacity all the time was a recipe for disaster, a rule that applies just as much to the National Health Service as it did to my small rural general practice. The UK government had certainly not learned this lesson in the years prior to the pandemic. While I understand that it is politically challenging to allocate funds for something that might not happen, we have since March 2020 learned the appalling impact of failing to prepare.

As Sir Simon Stevens, then chief executive of the NHS, told the Parliamentary Health and Social Care Committee in early 2021:

> Should we try to build more resilience into public services rather than running everything to the optimum just-in-time efficiency? I think that is one of the big lessons from the pandemic ... Resilience requires buffer, and buffer can look wasteful until the moment when it is not.[9]

The LSE–Lancet Commission on the future of the NHS clearly showed that public spending on health has consistently been lower in the UK than in most other high-income countries. At a time of increasing need, spending on social care has decreased in real terms, and most other wealthy countries spend more than us. Furthermore, after decades of improvement, increases in life expectancy have begun to slow, and for males they have even started to go into reverse.[10] We clearly have plenty of catching up to do.

Preparing for the future
But there are ways of preparing for the future besides simply increasing spending. The remarkable success of the Covid vaccination programme, both in the UK and elsewhere, has brought renewed attention to the immense value of prevention, while the example of the UK's Nightingale hospitals beautifully demonstrates an important aspect of modern healthcare. Simply providing more hospital beds is rarely the whole answer – unless, of course, a lack of hospital capacity happens to be the problem.

If, as seems clear, there is never going to be enough money, how do we go about making choices? What is the real intended value of healthcare, and what is the best possible outcome? After all, disease and infirmity will never disappear completely, so how can we ensure that we are using the funds available in the best possible way?

Once the immediate challenge of recovering from the pandemic has been addressed, we should start to anticipate future problems – and it is clear that simply spending more money year after year is unlikely to be the sole solution. As we look beyond a world dominated by Covid-19, we must ask two critical questions. What is healthcare? And what is it for?

While these questions might seem straightforward, there are certainly no simple answers. In all too many countries, there is little clarity about what healthcare systems are ultimately *for* and what they are trying to achieve. And what are the limits – where might the boundaries of healthcare be? After all, if we don't know what we are trying to achieve, how can we ever budget for it? While many healthcare leaders develop impressive medium-term plans, their actual behaviours and choices in a crisis do not always seem to match their noble aspirations. In any other sphere of life, we would question the wisdom of pouring money into projects without strictly defined boundaries. This would be no more logical than trying to fill a bucket with a hole in the bottom – and about as effective.

Your answer to the question of what healthcare is for will inevitably depend on your personal perspective. A patient needing care or their loved one, for instance, will see things very differently from a doctor treating patients, a healthcare administrator delivering services or a policymaker planning services for the future. As someone who has worn all four hats, I know how challenging this can be.

As a patient

If you are a patient or their loved one, the question of what healthcare is for will probably seem relatively straightforward. You will naturally want everything that can be offered to make and keep you – or your relative or friend – fit and well with a long and active life. That doesn't seem too much to ask.

In late 2018, just after I'd started to plan this book, I found myself needing urgent and aggressive treatment for a form of head and neck cancer. This meant undergoing a couple of operations, followed by thirty sessions of radiotherapy and five of chemotherapy. At the end of my first bout of radiotherapy, as I sat up from the bench where I had been anchored in a claustrophobia-inducing plastic mesh mask under a massive radiotherapy machine, I recall thinking how lucky I was to be living in a country with a health service that meant that I didn't have to think about the cost of the treatment I was receiving, let alone pay for any of it. It felt extraordinary that other citizens had contributed towards the enormous cost of my care through their taxes, in the same way that I had contributed to the care of others. Cancer was quite worrying enough, without the added fear of bankruptcy. Indeed, the only personal costs that I faced during many months of treatment were for the fuel in my car for my journeys to the hospital and the parking costs when I got there, although research from Macmillan Cancer Relief in 2021 showed that around four in five people with cancer in the UK face additional living costs or a loss of income, amounting to an average of £891 a month on top of their usual spending.[11]

During my treatment, I was very aware that the medical care I was receiving was seriously expensive, and not just because of the drugs and radiotherapy. I was looked after by an extensive and skilled multi-disciplinary team of doctors, nurses, healthcare assistants, radiotherapists, physiotherapists, speech and language therapists, dentists, dental hygienists, audiologists, dieticians, receptionists and porters, as well as the behind-the scenes administrative, managerial and support staff who matter so much to the smooth running of any hospital.

In countries that don't have a universal healthcare system, the costs to the patient can be astronomical and are a leading cause of bankruptcy. We should remember when we are considering the cost of healthcare that it isn't just an abstract matter of academic interest – it can be central to personal questions of affluence and poverty, of life and death. This is a challenge that ultimately impacts on every one of us.

As a doctor

I worked as a doctor for nearly forty years – initially in hospitals and then as a general practitioner, dealing with the day-to-day challenges of life for a practice population in a rural area of the UK. I once calculated that in the course of my career I must have carried out about a quarter of a million consultations. In each and every one of them, my prime responsibility was to the individual patient.

Like all doctors, I was registered with the UK's General Medical Council, the body that maintains the official register of medical practitioners. The responsibility of the doctor to the individual patient in the GMC's key document, 'Good Medical Practice', could not be more clear. The first rule is: 'Make the care of your patient your first concern.'

However, if only life was quite that simple; the reality of life as a doctor is rather more nuanced. In another document titled 'Leadership and Management for All Doctors' the GMC has stressed that 'being a good doctor means more than simply being a good clinician', going on to advise its doctors to 'use resources efficiently for the benefit of patients and the public'.

What does this mean in practical terms? If I see a patient with a relatively trivial symptom that is causing them some annoyance without being in any way life-threatening, and the only treatment available is massively expensive, what should I do? If I refer them for treatment, am I failing in my commitment to 'use resources efficiently for the benefit of patients and the public'? But if I don't, am I choosing not to make the care of my patient my first concern? Would my decision be different if the patient was paying for their own treatment?

In my years as a family doctor, I regularly had to make such decisions, while considering issues such as the impact of referrals on waiting times. If GPs chose to refer every patient to hospital care where there was a chance it would be helpful, it is likely that the backlog of work generated would significantly reduce access for those who need it most. If I was a patient with a minor symptom, I might feel irritated at not being referred, but if I was a patient with a serious condition and my care was impacted by other people's less dangerous problems, I would almost certainly feel even more dismayed. In any system where funding is finite, trade-offs are inevitable. If we could be clearer about the most effective use of healthcare, we would all benefit.

As a healthcare administrator

For those involved in planning and administration, as I have been myself, these challenges become even more acute. People who run hospitals or are involved in the organization of a regional or national health service must make major trade-offs. Every day they must take decisions and make choices about the purchase of equipment, the availability of staff, how to find a balance between prevention and treatment, the number of beds that need to be available, the type of specialists that should be recruited, the staff-to-patient ratio and a great deal more.

As a simple example, if you are responsible for a large geographical area and need to offer the greatest benefit for the management of stroke, how do you share funding between prevention, diagnosis, the acute management of people who have already experienced a stroke and their long-term support? Although it is likely that the most dramatic new diagnostics and treatments will create headlines and offer the most obvious benefit, the funding of well-targeted and effective prevention might ultimately have more benefit. If you are running a private hospital that is reliant on attracting work to generate income, your investment might be straightforward. But if you are looking at the overall impact on an area, your choices might be very different, with prevention potentially becoming a more attractive option.

The problem with prevention is that it tends to be invisible. We almost never meet someone who is aware that prevention has helped them, because the whole point is that it stops something from happening. It is entirely possible that I have so far avoided a heart attack because of preventative advice I've been given by my doctor. However, as I'll never know for sure, there's nothing to celebrate. During the vaccination programme for the Covid-19 pandemic, we have begun to look at prevention differently, with its benefits finally visible to many people. The scale of the campaign, and the sense of safety it has brought, has made many of us appreciate the benefits of preventative healthcare. But in many other areas of medicine the situation is very different, with prevention regarded as the poor relation.

As a government
From a governmental perspective, healthcare is astonishingly expensive. In the early phases of the coronavirus pandemic, an

astronomical level of resource was required to keep the population safe. With a rapidly spreading and invisible but identifiable enemy, governments made sure the money could be found – at almost any cost. But in more normal times, the challenge doesn't disappear – far from it, in fact.

I spent over a decade working at a senior national level in the British NHS, culminating in six years as chair of NICE, the National Institute for Health and Care Excellence. Part of the role of the institute is to look at new and expensive technologies and treatments, in order to determine if they are cost-effective and should be used by the NHS. As a result, my experience extends from the truly personal – my own experience of cancer – through to the national and even the international. I was privileged to advise senior ministers in countries around the world, all of whom face the same extraordinary challenge of affording healthcare. And when I did, I would ask every one of them the same question, which I also posed in a session at the World Health Assembly in Geneva: 'Do you really know what your healthcare system is trying to achieve?'

If we examine our healthcare systems from a historical perspective, we find that many of them were introduced to ensure that a country had a sufficiently healthy workforce, or a sufficiently fit population to defend itself in case of war. However, as the possibilities offered by medicine and pharmaceuticals have expanded beyond all recognition, the activities on which money can be spent have become disconnected from these original aspirations.

If this feels a little abstract and theoretical, consider a 2019 report from the *Guardian* in which a clinical psychologist described loneliness as 'social isolation syndrome' and suggested that drugs might be developed to address the problem.[12] This is a remarkable idea, and I will repeat it here lest it seem implausible. This was a serious discussion in which medication was being proposed as a treatment for loneliness. I do not wish to undermine the importance of loneliness, to minimize the heartache it can cause or to disregard the strong correlations that exist with ill health. But what concerns me is the question of whether expanding the remit of therapeutic healthcare at a time when our healthcare systems are facing escalating costs is either logical or wise. The overmedicalization of everyday life has an inevitable impact on the systems' capacity. For instance, the recognition that obesity and a lack of physical fitness were risk factors that made the development of severe illness with Covid-19 more likely led Boris Johnson to announce that GPs would prescribe cycling.[13] The underlying idea – cycling is good for you – is excellent. However, the idea that doctors should be involved in *prescribing* this activity was symptomatic of an approach to healthcare that seems entirely unsustainable.

Ever-increasing costs and uncertain intentions are not the most logical of companions, as they can lead governments to pour good money after bad without being sure why. It is bad enough to have insufficient funds to treat all the disease and challenges we have already identified, but the situation will be many times worse if the wish list of healthcare keeps expanding.

What's it all for?
I am aware that my suggestion that we don't know what we want our healthcare to achieve might sound ridiculous, so let me explain. While I am sure that you knew exactly what you wanted from your own healthcare when you last went to see your GP or consulted another health professional, that's not quite the same thing as how we determine what we want the system as a whole to achieve, or where the health budget might best be spent.

Again, the coronavirus pandemic shone a light on this question. During the initial phase of that crisis, our healthcare system's primary aim was to stop people dying from Covid-19. The massive resources that were pumped into health services all around the world were spent to keep people breathing and to give their families hope. This clarity led to a rapid re-prioritization, with funds, staff and expertise being moved to where they might best address the pandemic. For a while, organ transplants were halted and even radiotherapy was deferred. Almost no aspect of our healthcare system was unaffected. But these were not normal times; as we negotiate a 'new normal', the challenging questions still have to be faced.

No healthcare system can be designed to deal with a pandemic, and nor should it be – that isn't its job. Although it must absolutely be ready to adapt to an emergency, it cannot possibly sit in a state of readiness for an event that is likely to happen no more frequently than once every few decades. It isn't feasible to have massive numbers of extra staff and beds waiting on the off-chance. Instead, we must plan for the everyday and have contingency plans for the unexpected.

In normal times, the role of healthcare systems is to deal with people's day-to-day needs – whether that is in community-based primary healthcare, including general practice, or in hospital. To use an analogy, these organizations are a little like lorries – fantastically effective and generally reliable, but very slow. In a pandemic, we need something agile – a suitable metaphor might be a Porsche. We would never expect a Porsche to do the job of a lorry, or vice versa. They are each perfectly designed to fulfil a particular role and poorly designed to do each other's.

In the same way, the pandemic required a fundamentally different type of healthcare system, with dramatically increased hospital capacity, fully staffed intensive care beds and a strict focus on dealing with the most acute and the most urgent problems – an entirely different expectation compared to the system we need in normal circumstances.

Away from a crisis, you might believe that every healthcare system is designed both to treat disease and to maintain and improve the health of its population. However, while this certainly sounds logical, if this really is the intended approach, why would we not invest more in prevention, in understanding the causes of ill health and in education – in *health* rather than healthcare?

Health versus healthcare

I am well aware that a healthy population is likely to be a productive population, which might mean that high-quality healthcare could conceivably be seen as self-financing. However, at present, this feels more like theory than reality. Even prior to Covid-19, the proportion of GDP spent on health in most countries was increasing. And while the underfunding of healthcare has long been an issue, it does not automatically follow that simply providing more money is the only solution.

Although they are related, health and healthcare are in no way the same thing. The Institute for Healthcare Improvement has described the fundamental purpose of healthcare as being 'to enhance quality of life by enhancing health'. Nevertheless, when funding has been reduced and money is tight, cuts tend to be made in the same areas. Preventative healthcare and public health may be spoken of as being a genuine priority, but the behaviour of governments around the world suggests the opposite. As an example, the US spends just 2.5 per cent of its healthcare budget on public health. In spring 2020, at the onset of the Covid-19 pandemic, underfunded health departments were struggling to deal with an epidemic in opioid addiction, climbing obesity rates, contaminated water and easily preventable diseases.[14]

The situation is, of course, immensely complex. How do we ever begin to balance the vast sums that can be spent on a single seriously ill patient against the distressing conditions in which many frail and elderly people live out their final years, often as a result of a lack of adequate funding?

In 2015, the *Daily Telegraph* reported that the price of a single year's treatment of a drug called eculizumab, developed to treat a rare type of blood disease called paroxysmal nocturnal haemoglobinuria, was £340,000 per patient, which would mean a total lifetime cost of around £10 million for each sufferer.[15] In 2019, the US Food and Drug Administration approved what was at the time the most expensive drug in the world, a gene therapy developed by the Swiss multinational pharmaceutical corporation Novartis that treats spinal muscular atrophy at a cost of $2.1 million per patient.[16] The price of this drug, which has the brand name Zolgensma, is more than double that of the world's second most expensive drug, an $850,000 treatment for blindness called Luxturna. In March 2021, Zolgensma was made available on the British NHS at a price that was described as 'fair to taxpayers', following a confidential deal struck by NHS England.[17]

The more we understand the potential of new technologies such as genomics and personalized medicine, the higher these healthcare costs may become. Fantastic new possibilities are emerging as approaches such as whole genome sequencing, the increasing use of data and informatics and wearable technology move us to an era of truly personalized care. These treatments are tailored to the needs of the individual patient, but they are also mind-blowingly expensive.

The societal impact of such innovation might be profound. If we can't afford these massively expensive drugs for everyone who needs them – and we almost certainly can't – then how will we decide who will get them? If they end up being reserved for the rich, we will have a major ethical and political problem.

It is generally accepted that increasing social inequality is causing real problems; the mega-rich are becoming wealthier, but the trickle-down effect to everyone else's incomes that many people predicted does not appear to have materialized. It doesn't take much imagination to picture a world in which a tiny elite can receive these expensive drugs and consequently survive diseases that are fatal to everyone else. It is also easy to imagine the anger and unrest that would result from such inequality – history will judge us on how we make these decisions.

Even today, although we choose to fund a handful of exceptionally expensive drugs, some patients find themselves having to endure lengthy waits for painful conditions, while others receive no treatment at all. In 2018, well before the pandemic, a survey by an independent think tank revealed that 80 per cent of NHS finance directors in England believed that funding pressures had caused people in need of mental health treatment to wait longer for care.[18] The problem is not simply that we need to spend more money on healthcare, at a time when every projection shows costs rising inexorably. The challenge that we are facing is particularly demanding because of the difficult practical and ethical questions that it raises. How can we decide whether it is preferable to spend healthcare funding on a single person with a rare, serious and hugely expensive condition, or 1,000 people with common and cheap but painful conditions? These are complex areas, packed with ethical dilemmas that become more important as costs escalate.

More money?
Any discussion on healthcare spending tends to trigger the usual demand that governments should simply spend more money. But while this is never sufficient on its own – at least in the long term – this is not to say that governmental budgeting has always got it right. The austerity politics of British prime minister David Cameron and his chancellor George Osborne in the wake of the global financial crisis left the National Health Service under-resourced, under-staffed and woefully under-prepared for the challenges that it would face, particularly during the pandemic. However, simply 'increasing the money' is not a long-term solution, at least not if we don't also address the issues of purpose, function, distribution and aspiration.

For the populations of countries that rely on individual funding or insurance for healthcare, the issue of how public money should be spent may not seem relevant. However, as their costs and insurance premiums spiral, how can they tell whether the expense is justified? Is the expensive operation that they might have been offered really the most effective solution to their problem? And who should they trust when they want to find out? After all, however affluent the country you live in, healthcare is a scarce resource, which means that it is rationed. The simple fact is that demand for healthcare is almost infinite, and funding never can be. Decisions have to be made – and the key thing is to do this rationally.

In the US, most healthcare is privately financed, and so most decisions on rationing come down to price: you get what you – or your employer – can afford to insure you for. But this also has implications for public finance. The current system of employer-financed health insurance is only able to thrive because the American government makes the premiums tax-deductible, which has been calculated to equate to a healthcare subsidy of more than $200 billion. If you are a US citizen, that's your money being spent.

For US citizens who are without health insurance and depend on public sector care, healthcare is characterized by long waits, high patient co-payments, low salaries for doctors and limits on payments to hospitals. Some people's care will be rationed simply because they run out of money. It is critical that every healthcare system in the world finds safe, equitable ways of distributing their resources, and many of them could be much more effective.

For instance, a 2019 report concluded that of every $4 spent on healthcare in the United States, as much as $1 may be wasted, due to a combination of administrative complexity, failures in the coordination and delivery of services, overtreatment or low-value care, pricing failure and fraud.[19] William Shrank, the chief medical officer at the American health insurance company Humana and the author of the study, estimated that the total annual cost of waste in the US healthcare system was between $760 billion and $935 billion, more than the total economic output of Turkey. In that year, it was estimated that $3.82 trillion would be spent on healthcare in the United States, of which almost 25 per cent was wasted. Clarity as to the aim of all this care would make an immense difference, but it is based on activity rather than outcomes. And while eliminating waste can make a very real difference, it in no way answers the challenge of perpetually increasing costs.

In countries around the world, research is being undertaken into the concept of low-value care, typically defined as an intervention where evidence suggests it confers little or no benefit on patients, where the risk of harm exceeds the likely benefit or, more broadly, where the costs of the intervention do not provide proportional added benefits.[20] Have you ever considered that such treatments might exist?

WE'VE GOT A PROBLEM

Doesn't it seem extraordinary that modern healthcare might offer treatments that carry a risk of doing more harm than good?

Observing where healthcare funding is spent can give us a clue to a country's priorities. To generalize, modern medical science is pouring more and more money into the aggressive treatment of the seriously ill, as exemplified by the idea of 'one more course' of chemotherapy in people who are close to death. Is this always logical? Is this what society truly wants? If we are trying to beat death, it's a game that we will inevitably lose. However, these are not simple questions. It is all well and good to say that we should prioritize prevention, until you or your loved one has the aggressive cancer. And your priorities may well change if it is your parent who has dementia, and their final months and years will cause your entire family a great deal of distress. We might find that what we want for ourselves is different from what we want for the whole of society. So how do we handle that?

After all, healthcare is hugely expensive. Every single action carried out by a nurse, a doctor or a therapist costs money. In countries without universal healthcare, this is a tangible cost that must be directly paid by the patient or through an insurance scheme. In the UK, we rarely think about the cost from a personal perspective – it simply isn't on our agenda. Apart from a few exceptions, such as prescription fees, dental fees and the irritation of having to pay for parking during hospital trips, our care feels as if it is entirely free, but this is not the case. When your taxes are used to pay the bills, it is your money that is being spent.

Whether the costs are covered by individuals or the state, money is never going to be limitless – at least in non-pandemic times. And unless we take some tough decisions, it is inevitable that at some point there simply won't be enough money to pay for all the healthcare that we want or feel that we need. Indeed, the situation is even worse than that – in what might seem a rather perverse trend, the more nations spend on healthcare, the more it costs. The 1942 Beveridge Report, which led to the establishment of the National Health Service in the UK, predicted that costs would fall as the population became healthier. It stated that a comprehensive health service would 'diminish disease by prevention and cure' and that costs would subsequently stabilize. In reality, of course, the reverse turned out to be the case. In the UK, health spending per head rose from £9 per annum in 1949–50 to £2,187 in 2016–17.[21] Even allowing for inflation, these are astonishing figures. In 1949–50, UK health spending was 3.5 per cent of GDP; by 2016–17 it had more than doubled, to 7.3 per cent. And these are not just theoretical figures – they refer to the real spending of real money.

In 2013, the distinguished British health economist Professor John Appleby wrote: 'If the next fifty years follow the trajectory of the past fifty, then the United Kingdom could be spending nearly one-fifth of its entire wealth on the public provision of health and social care.'[22] Later in the paper he continued, 'If healthcare spending were to grow at the rate seen over the decade since 1999–2000, however, then by the mid-2070s the NHS would be consuming close to 100 per cent of GDP. Clearly this is not a fiscally sustainable trend.'

It certainly isn't, and this is far from just a British phenomenon. In the US, the Congressional Budget Office carried out an analysis in 2007 detailing projections of federal and national spending on healthcare over a seventy-five-year period to 2082.[23] Assuming that there was no change to the historic rate of excess costs, their projections estimated that healthcare spending would take up 33.3 per cent of GDP by 2035 and 98.9 per cent by 2082. This would leave a mere 1.1 per cent of GDP to pay for defence, education, infrastructure and everything else.

Just like all predictions, however, this will turn out to be wrong. There have already been significant changes in US healthcare spending since that report was written, and future predictions will no doubt give different percentages. But the message will be the same: spending is going up. And this trend is global.

A 2018 paper in *The Lancet* examined global trends in spending by looking at historical health financing data for 188 countries from 1995 to 2015.[24] The authors then estimated future scenarios of health spending for the next two decades. Global health spending was projected to increase from $10 trillion in 2015 to $20 trillion in 2040. If you find the idea of a trillion dollars hard to conceptualize, it is $1,000,000,000,000 (or about £786,800,000,000). The trouble with such big numbers is that they end up being almost completely meaningless. Most of us can't help but glaze over when economists talk about these huge figures, but they represent real, spendable money, with real costs that impact on real people.

In countries where individuals are responsible for paying for their own care, the challenge of finding sufficient funds becomes more acute. An article in the *New York Times* told the story of Carrie Cota, a fifty-six-year-old travel agent from California, who was diagnosed with the autoimmune disease lupus erythematosus in 2007.[25] She ran up thousands of dollars in medical and dental bills and ended up losing her job and her house. Another American report revealed that huge numbers of people struggle with the cost of long-term conditions like diabetes, which cost sufferers an average of $26,971 per year, and neurological disorders like multiple sclerosis, which cost an average of $34,167 per year. The biggest expense was hospitalization, which in many cases resulted in bankruptcy.[26]

Furthermore, these costs are escalating all the time. A 2015 study by the US National Bureau of Economic Research showed that the prices of cancer drugs increased by 10 per cent every year between 1995 and 2013. Again, this is the sort of statistic that we might gloss over with a stifled yawn, but we should remember that this is real money, with real year-on-year increases – and that it impacts on real human beings, with real cancers. In the UK, hospital spending on drugs rose at an average rate of 12.1 per cent a year between 2010–11 and 2016–17, from around £4.2 billion to £8.3 billion.[27] The British NHS issued 25 million prescriptions in 1949. By 2016, this had increased to 1.3 billion – a fifty-fold increase. In a population of 65 million citizens, that equates to twenty prescriptions per person per year. For what it's worth, I personally receive prescriptions for four different therapies every month. Of course, I think I'm worth it – but then I would say that, wouldn't I? Is everybody else worth it too? Yes, of course they are, but how do we pay?

In the UK, even though most healthcare costs are covered by the National Health Service, expense can still be a major issue – both for individuals who may face anxiety about whether effective care will be available and for the taxpayers who have to pay for it. A 2016 report from Cancer Research UK expressed concern that cancer treatment is becoming unsustainable, stating that 'healthcare systems around the globe, including the NHS, are struggling to afford cancer drugs'.[28] It continued:

> There are no signs that this trend for hefty price tags will abate any time soon or that these prices can be easily reined in. There is concern around where these prices are heading and the implications on cancer treatment, and

healthcare in general in light of financially constrained healthcare systems.

Choosing the best

When you and I are considering purchasing something, we generally consider the cost, the quality and the state of our finances. We might dream of a top-of-the-range BMW, but after consideration choose a car that is more compatible with what we can afford. Regardless of what we're purchasing – a phone, a holiday, a computer – the process is the same. We look at the products available and consider what we can afford, before usually making some kind of compromise.

When it comes to our health, the rules of the game appear to be very different. When we receive a life-changing diagnosis, we simply want the best care. In the UK, we don't have to consider what we can personally afford, but in many countries this is a major aspect of the challenge of serious illness – and even this isn't straightforward. Can we assume that the most expensive treatment is the best? Would we be risking our lives if we were to choose a cheaper option? And could we ever forgive ourselves if we made the wrong choice?

Indeed, when it comes to health, the concept of choice is hugely complex. In most aspects of life, we are able to make choices based on how highly we value something. The same item of clothing can vary in price, determined by such issues as the quality of material, the quality of manufacturing, design, fashion and brand. If we want to buy a pair of jeans, for instance, we make a judgement based on how much these variables matter to us.

But in healthcare, the same principles do not apply. Back in 1963, the economist Kenneth Arrow wrote a paper titled 'Uncertainty and the Welfare Economics of Medical Care',[29] in which he highlighted key differences with the choice model that we use elsewhere. We can't test out the product before we purchase it, it is difficult to change our minds later and we know that we may ultimately pay for making the wrong choice with our lives. To cap it all, we will know far less about the benefits and risks than the doctor treating us, and we might feel that we just have to trust them. Most of the time we will be right to do so, but the usual laws of economics don't appear to apply – and they certainly don't help to keep prices down.

Even in a country such as the UK, where individual citizens don't have to pay for their care directly, we simply can't afford everything. I can't begin to formulate a way of working out what 'everything for everyone' would cost, but it is not inconceivable that it would exceed our GDP. Indeed, as I will show, every successful treatment tends to lead to further expenditure, so we must make some difficult choices.

There is something deeply uncomfortable about the thought that the benefits of some healthcare are not worth the expense. When we are considering the health of a loved one, none of us would feel comfortable in deciding that a level of care or treatment is too expensive to be worthwhile. 'How can you possibly put a price on life?' is an oft-asked question, but when the costs of care become astronomically high, these challenges have to be faced. My family is worth the world to me. I'd be more than happy for the whole of the UK's GDP to be spent on keeping them healthy, but in a system where we share the risks and the costs, the question is, how much would I be prepared for the state to spend not on my family but on *your* family, your next-door neighbour's family or the homeless man you pass in the street? When the personnel involved are different, the ethical considerations become almost immeasurable, but these costs can be huge. According to Jennifer Kent, the head of California's state Department of Health Care Services, the medical expenses of a single child in the state totalled $21 million in one year.[30]

No country is immune to these problems. A few years ago, I met Dr Ulana Suprun, who was then Ukraine's minister of health, having previously practised as a radiologist in Michigan and New York. In an interview in *The Lancet*, she said, 'It was [an] extremely inefficient [system] in Ukraine … Every year, 680,000 families go bankrupt because they have to pay for the healthcare of their loved one … They live in fear of going to the doctor. 23 per cent of patients last year said that they did not even go to the doctor when they became ill because they were afraid they [the doctors] would diagnose something serious.'[31]

All around the world, prices continue to spiral. According to the American Institute of Cancer Research, cancer costs the world about $895 billion a year – more than any other disease. Alongside drugs, that includes the costs of diagnosis, radiotherapy, imaging, pathology, surgery and end-of-life care. And in many countries, for most of the population, the care that cancer patients receive is minimal. If everyone who needed treatment was able to get it, the potential costs could be astronomical – and they would be unaffordable for many countries.

Faced with impossibly complex problems like these, we can generally choose to either solve them or ignore them. In the world of politics, there is a temptation to ignore complex dilemmas in the hope that they become the responsibility of your successor, leaving someone else to make the decisions or take the blame. There will never be enough money to pay for all the healthcare that people want. Disease and infirmity will never disappear completely. So how do we decide how much healthcare is enough?

How much is enough?

Before we can even begin to find a solution, we need to understand what is going on. I've been a doctor for nearly fifty years, and so I inevitably think like one. The first step in treating any type of problem has to be reaching a diagnosis – only then can we hope to find a cure.

As an example, and as an appropriate analogy for healthcare funding, consider the medical problem of anaemia, defined as a condition in which there is a deficiency of red blood cells or haemoglobin in the blood. Anaemia is typically diagnosed with a simple blood test, but this doesn't tell us anything about the cause. It is just a description – just as healthcare systems having insufficient resources is simply a description.

When confronted with anaemia, student doctors are taught to think logically. If there is insufficient haemoglobin in the bloodstream, it is likely that either not enough haemoglobin is being made or that enough is made but even more is being lost. These two possibilities can be sub-divided further. For instance, not enough may be made because the patient is not eating the right nutrients or because these nutrients aren't being absorbed from the gut. Haemoglobin may be lost because of bleeding or because the red blood cells are being broken down. Inherited or autoimmune disorders and infections such as malaria and septicaemia can decrease their lifespan, while periods of rapid growth or high energy requirements, such as puberty or pregnancy, may cause demand to exceed supply.

If there is bleeding, this could be coming from numerous places. If it is coming from the stomach, this may be caused by a cancer or an ulcer, or it might be a side effect of medication. Diagnosing anaemia is simply the start of the process.

'So what?' you may be thinking. 'How is any of this relevant?' Well, you can only begin to treat a problem when you understand what is causing it. For instance, if a poor dietary intake is the cause of anaemia, giving iron supplements may treat it successfully, but the same supplements will be useless if the cause is internal bleeding.

It is just the same if you are trying to treat an apparent shortage of healthcare funding – an anaemic healthcare system. If you fail to understand the cause of the challenge, you risk pouring more funds in while getting no lasting benefit. Opposition politicians often demand that more money be spent, but that may not always be the correct answer – although that doesn't stop it being a popular, simple and easy-to-explain approach.

At the risk of being as simplistic in addressing this challenge as I've been in my description of the treatment of anaemia, the possible causes of the gap between the funding available for healthcare and the demands placed on the system might include any of the following:

- Insufficient funds are being provided or demand is rising faster than spending
- Sufficient funds are provided, but funding is being wasted
- Funding is aimed at the wrong area of care
- Priorities are skewed, leading some conditions to receive more funding than others
- Healthcare industries repeatedly create demand for the treatment of conditions that were previously unrecognized and untreated

This book will attempt to unravel some of the possible causes of this challenge, which faces every country on earth, before assessing some possible solutions. I concede that if there was a simple solution, we would have found it long ago, but I do know one thing with absolute certainty: we cannot ignore this problem any longer.

Our society can choose to spend more on healthcare, but this will mean spending less on other things – on education, roads and bridges, security and defence. If we choose *not* to spend more, we could instead choose to limit people's behaviours that we think are bad for their health, in an attempt to reduce costs. In the Covid-19 pandemic, when populations went into lockdown and restrictions on travel and interacting were introduced, people's health did improve – but in only one way. The effects on other aspects of health were considerable.

Indeed, the impact of Covid-19 on our healthcare systems is becoming increasingly clear. Because there were many months when treatment that was not related to Covid was significantly reduced, many cancers went undiagnosed and untreated, mental health problems escalated and screening programmes ground to a halt. To illustrate the point, in the UK, some 46,000 fewer patients started treatment for cancer between April 2020 and February 2021 compared to the previous year.

Internationally, the impact of Covid-19 on healthcare has been massive. For instance, an estimated 1.4 million fewer people received care for tuberculosis in 2020 than in 2019, according to data compiled by the World Health Organization. The countries with the biggest relative gaps were Indonesia, South Africa, the Philippines and India. As Dr Tedros Adhanom Ghebreyesus, director general of the World Health Organization, made clear,

'The effects of COVID-19 go far beyond the death and disease caused by the virus itself.'[32]

The challenges facing every healthcare system are huge. Even before Covid-19, escalating demand and cost were rendering them unsustainable. I don't intend to ask here how we should pay for care or what proportion of a nation's GDP should be spent on it, though I will briefly assess some of the options. I don't want to debate the benefits of general taxation, hypothecated taxation or insurance, but I do want to ask the key questions. How do we know what is good value and what is cost-effective? Why are the costs of healthcare constantly escalating? How do we decide what we can afford? And most importantly, what do we want from it?

In 1959, the biologist René Dubos wrote a book called *Mirage of Health*, in which he pointed out that 'complete and lasting freedom from disease is but a dream remembered from imaginings of a Garden of Eden'.[33] Is that a fair reflection of what we are trying to achieve? None of these are small questions, and there aren't easy answers, but it should certainly be interesting.

CHAPTER 2

How Did We Get Here?

At first glance, it all seems rather curious – because we should be winning.

Year on year, science has made consistent improvements, and medical research is able to answer increasingly complex questions about sickness and health, progress that has had a particular impact on how long we can expect to live. Estimates suggest that in a pre-Enlightenment world, global life expectancy was around thirty years, largely because of dreadful levels of infant mortality. However, by the early nineteenth century, people in industrialized countries were starting to live longer. And since 1900, the global life expectancy has more than doubled and is now approaching seventy.

It has been calculated that global life expectancy improved as much during the twentieth century as it had done in the preceding 8,000 years. Today, it is higher even in the poorest countries than it was in the developed nations in 1800. Every nation is doing better than the previous best, an astonishing achievement for humanity.

In 1948, the year that the British National Health Service was founded, the UK average life expectancy was 65.9 years for men and 70.3 for women. I was born just after the birth of the NHS. Before this time, I would have been considered lucky to have lived to my current age. By 2016, life expectancy had increased by about thirteen years, to 79.5 for men and 83.1 for women. All around the world, the changes have been remarkable. In the Caribbean, life expectancy in 1950 was just fifty-one; by 2015, it had risen to seventy-three. And in the continent of Africa, life expectancy in 1950 was a mere thirty-six; by 2015 it had nearly doubled, to sixty-one.

However, and against the global pattern, changes can still vary significantly year on year. For instance, in 2015, life expectancy fell across most of Europe. In England, life expectancy fell by 0.2 years in both males and females following an estimated 28,000 deaths associated with flu, a change that was unprecedented for decades until the Covid pandemic hit in early 2020.[1] Covid itself has had a profound impact. A report from Oxford University in 2021 showed that life expectancy for both men and women was reduced by over a year, wiping out the improvements of the previous decade.[2]

Despite this recent blip, humanity has much to be proud about – although we should never forget the massive negative impact of poverty and inequality. Life expectancy varies hugely between countries – Japan's is currently double that of Sierra Leone – and there are also entirely unacceptable variations within countries. It has been calculated that the average life expectancy for someone born in London drops by one year for every two stops that you travel eastward on a London Underground train from Westminster on the Jubilee Line.[3] Alternatively, if you travel eastbound from Lancaster Gate to Mile End – twenty minutes on the Central Line – life expectancy decreases by an astonishing twelve years. This change is primarily associated with decreasing affluence; a study in the US revealed that those American men whose income is in the top 1 per cent live fifteen years longer than those in the poorest 1 per cent; for women, the gap is ten years.[4]

Covid has had a massive impact in these deprivation variabilities, too. While data published by the Office of National Statistics suggests that the most deprived areas of England have twice the rate of deaths involving Covid-19 than the most affluent, it is clear that this is not simply an effect of Covid-19.[5]

Inequalities in mortality have long been evident across many causes of death. Indeed, deaths from suicide, conditions such as liver disease and cancer as well as overall mortality rates all show that death rates for people living in the most deprived decile of the country are higher than those in the least deprived.[6]

A short time prior to the pandemic, Sir Michael Marmot, director of the UCL Institute of Health Equity, published research that linked austerity measures in the UK to the country's first fall in life expectancy for more than a century. His report showed that for about a century before 2010, life expectancy in Britain had improved by about one year every four years.[7] In men, it had risen from 79.01 years in 2010–12 to 79.56 years in 2016–18, while for women it increased from 82.83 to 83.18 in the same period. The largest increases in life expectancy were in the least deprived 10 per cent of neighbourhoods in London, but in the most deprived areas in the north-east of England, women's life expectancy had dropped from 77.64 to 76.79.

Why is this likely to have occurred? Falling expenditure on public services is almost certainly the key. In 2009–10, public sector expenditure was 42 per cent of GDP, but by 2018–19 it had fallen to 35 per cent. Although the life expectancy of wealthier people continued to increase, it stagnated or even declined for the poorest citizens in the north. Marmot's report demonstrated that at least 80 per cent of the change in life expectancy between 2011 and 2019 was a result of influences other than winter-associated mortality, the explanation provided by the government. It also showed that the slowing of life expectancy improvement in the UK was more marked than in most European and other high-income countries, except the US.

A subsequent report on the impact of Covid showed that life expectancy in north-west England fell in 2020 by 1.6 years for men and 1.2 years for women, compared with 1.3 years and 0.9 years across England as a whole.[8] And within the region, life expectancy dipped most sharply in areas characterized by poverty and deprivation.

As I will stress repeatedly in this book, our health isn't simply a matter of how much money is spent on healthcare. Because it is so closely linked to the circumstances in which we are born, grow, live, work and age, it is inevitable that funding cuts will have an adverse effect. The more deprived the area, the lower the life expectancy.

It is also vital to remember that historic life expectancy statistics are considerably skewed by high rates of infant mortality. One of the reasons that life expectancy as an average was so low in the distant past was because so many babies and children died in infancy. If the average life expectancy in a given era was forty-five, this did not mean that everyone was at risk of dropping dead at that age. If you survived infancy, you had a reasonable chance of living to a fairly old age – as a glance around any graveyard will tell you. What has changed dramatically, however, is that reaching old age is now much more common, while the improvements in childhood mortality have been remarkable. Globally, in the year that I was born, nearly one quarter of all children died before the age of five; now there are fewer than forty deaths for every thousand births. Immunization has played a massive part – for instance, the lives of an estimated 20 million children were saved through immunization against measles between 2000 and 2016 alone.[9] And as a specific example of progress, as recently as 1983 the average lifespan of a person with Down's syndrome was just twenty-five years. Today it is approximately sixty – more than double.[10]

The cost of care

Despite our long-term global achievements – or more likely as a side effect of them – the cost of healthcare keeps escalating. The global health economy went from being 8 per cent of the world's GDP to 8.6 per cent between 2000 and 2005. In absolute terms, adjusted for inflation, this represents a 35 per cent growth in health expenditure in just five years.

In most areas of life, improved technology leads to price reductions. Advances in agricultural science, for instance, have caused the cost of food production to fall, meaning that people can be fed more cheaply and efficiently.[11,12,13] It's the same with information technology, so what is it that makes healthcare so different? After all, the diseases that challenged clinicians in the distant past have almost all been defeated, and yet doctors are as busy as they ever have been – if not busier.

How does that make sense? Why aren't costs falling, like they tend to in every other sector? There appear to be three main factors: changing population demographics, inflation and income growth effect, and an increase in the intensity of clinical practice and innovation.

The Office for Budget Responsibility in the UK has concluded that the prime driver of rising healthcare costs is the increase in the intensity of clinical practice. Doctors do more, probably not just because it can be beneficial but because they can.

In my long career as a doctor, I've witnessed much of this change, some of which has been astonishing. We don't just find a solution to a problem, implement it and reap the rewards. We keep researching, we keep changing. We are never satisfied. That's science, and that's the way it should be.

———

My first ever job as a qualified doctor was as a house physician at the Warneford Hospital in Leamington Spa. The hospital has now been demolished to make way for a housing estate, but my memories of it remain vivid. The hours were long, the patients were varied and the science was frequently hopelessly flawed – not that we realized it at the time, of course. We thought – just as doctors practising today think – that we were at the cutting edge of modern medicine, and we had got it right. We were doing our best.

Back in the early 1970s, we thought peptic ulcers were caused by stress, and we treated sufferers with a combination of either barbiturate or benzodiazepine tranquillizers, psychotherapy, a fish and milk diet and antacids. People who were admitted with heart attacks were kept on strict bed rest for three weeks and were forbidden from doing so much as walking to the toilet, instead having to suffer the indignity of the bedpan. Indeed, not every patient who had suffered a heart attack was even admitted to hospital – before the advent of coronary care units, there was little evidence that admission helped. For similar reasons, most patients who had strokes were typically not taken to hospital – 'nothing could be done' and their admission seemed both unkind and futile. The patient would generally be left at home while relatives and the doctor awaited the often-inevitable outcome.

One doctor's career span later, and almost everything about those scenarios has changed beyond all recognition. We now know that most peptic ulcers, rather than being caused by stress or diet, are linked to infection by bacteria known as Helicobacter pylori. They typically respond to a cocktail of antibiotics and proton pump inhibitors (drugs that reduce the production of stomach acid), while tranquillizers, psychotherapy, and milk and fish diets are no longer part of routine treatment.

The treatment of heart attack has also changed fundamentally. Rather than being kept on strict bed rest, victims now receive urgent hospitalization and intensive treatment, followed by rapid mobilization – prolonged immobility is now known to be hugely dangerous. Three weeks of bed rest has become a second-day referral to the gym, an astonishing change.

I still have a heartfelt thank you letter from the family of one heart attack victim whom I treated way back in 1972. They wrote that they were intensely grateful to me and my colleagues for the care that had 'saved his life', but we now know that he was lucky to have survived the treatment, let alone the heart attack. The bed rest that we had so confidently insisted on was the perfect recipe for a blood clot that could have spread to the lungs and killed him, but we simply didn't know that at the time. I learned long ago that recovery and gratitude are not necessarily evidence of effective treatment.

Practitioners – and especially complementary practitioners – who proudly present piles of thank you letters as 'evidence' that their treatments must be effective need to be aware of this. The fact that many patients I treated during my career received therapies that have now been proven to be ineffective doesn't mean that my doctoring didn't help – I was doing my best, and I hope I was treating the patients with kindness and compassion – but the research is clear that many of the actual therapies were, at best, an irrelevance. The science keeps improving. While many treatments are now much more effective than they were, future research will no doubt show that some of today's beliefs are just as wrong as the therapies we used in the 1970s.

When it comes to treating strokes, changing protocols of care have had a huge impact. Best practice guidelines now state that 'patients presenting with acute symptoms should be immediately transferred to hospital for accurate diagnosis of stroke type, and urgent initiation of appropriate treatment'.[14] In 2005, the National Audit Office in the UK published a study showing that this guidance was not being followed, prompting a national strategy for stroke care. The subsequent recommendations not only helped improve outcomes for stroke patients through faster access to tests and treatment, but the associated efficiencies helped save the NHS an estimated £456 million between 2007–8 and 2013–14.[15]

Medical practice changes all the time, and it needs to – sometimes fundamentally. I realize that it can be frustrating for the general public – I recently heard a caller to a radio phone-in about dietary research plead, 'Why can't the scientists just make their minds up?' – but the glory and the challenge of science is that nothing is forever. Every new development and theory is tested and improved on, and thus progress is maintained. What may be an unsolvable challenge to one generation becomes routine for the next. However, as seems inevitable, the cost of success goes up and up. Progress is generally a wonderful, life-affirming thing, but it's rarely cheap.

I find it hard to believe, but the first ever video recorder that I purchased, many years ago, was priced at nearly £800. Its VHS technology produced recordings that felt magical at the time but now seem barely watchable, rather like peering through a snowstorm. Allowing for inflation, the equivalent price today would be well over £2,000, and yet a combination of technological development and plummeting prices mean that you can today buy a high-definition

Freeview set-top box with a personal video recorder and an electronic programme guide for less than £40.

An astonishing price reduction has coincided with a dramatic increase in quality, but this is rarely the trajectory in the cost of medical treatments or equipment, with the rare exception where a simple medication renders complex surgery unnecessary. The invention of the H2 antagonist drugs and proton pump inhibitors to manage peptic ulcers, followed by the recognition that treating Helicobacter infection could frequently be curative, effectively wiped out an entire specialty of surgery. Surgeons who practised increasingly sophisticated operations to treat peptic ulcers found themselves redundant almost overnight and had to find a different focus for their skills.[16] This, however, was a rare occurrence. Generally, costs go up and up – a topic we will return to later.

Constantly changing

The history of medicine hasn't been a simple story of continuous improvement. Many of the diseases that challenged doctors 200 years ago are now history, and a majority of the conditions suffered by patients a century ago have also been eliminated. Despite this, hospitals and doctors remain as busy as ever. While policymakers frequently see the future as an extension of the past, major changes can render entire approaches out of date. What worked as an approach for one era may be entirely inappropriate for the next, and that has a major impact on the delivery of healthcare.

In 1900, the three most common causes of death were pneumonia, tuberculosis and diarrhoea. Today, prior to the Covid-19 pandemic, the three most common are heart disease, cancer and respiratory disease. In 1900, heart disease killed 137 people per 100,000 per year. Today, that figure is 193 people, an apparent 40 per cent increase, but one of the chief reasons is that in the past, other conditions killed people before they could die of heart disease. As we prevent heart disease, more people survive long enough to develop cancer or dementia. If you solve one problem, you will inevitably be faced by another. We should always celebrate and be immensely thankful for the many improvements in healthcare. I couldn't be more grateful that effective care means that I have lived a decade longer than my dad. But we do need to face up to the ongoing implications, planning and making decisions accordingly. To do otherwise is to hide our heads in the sand.

If we are to understand how we have arrived at our current problems and consider how we might address them, it is crucial that we study the major shifts in modern healthcare delivery. In the early 1900s, medicine was generally – to quote the great British physician Sir Cyril Chantler – 'simple, ineffective and relatively safe', but, as he continued, 'it is now complex, effective and potentially dangerous'.[17] While past treatments were frequently useless, they had the great benefit of being cheap. My father was a family doctor in the 1950s and I recall him prescribing 'tonics' such as Mist Gentian Alkaline and an assortment of different-coloured placebos – harmless, but also useless. Since the Second World War, and particularly over the past thirty years or so, healthcare has become increasingly complex, involving many more professionals, and the cost has risen inexorably. At the same time, populations have become more aware of what care might be available, and less happy when it is not. Increasing complexity, increasing cost and increasing expectations are all signs of success, but they have created a massive side effect. How do we pay for it all?

To take a simplified historical perspective, if you consider the past century and a half, you can detect shifts in approach every fifty years or so. Until the 1950s, the majority of the greatest day-to-day healthcare challenges came from infectious disease. Public health measures became increasingly important, with populations facing the ravages of smallpox, cholera, influenza, tuberculosis and multiple other epidemics. In a single week in 1849, 3,183 deaths were reported in London, primarily from such conditions.[18] In *The Beloved Physician*, a biography of the famous late-nineteenth-century physician Sir James Mackenzie,[19] the author describes a day's work in Mackenzie's general practice. As well as coping with a flood of minor problems that he could not diagnose – something that all family doctors will still recognize – his working day involved dealing with conditions such as pneumonia, diphtheria, cholera and acute rheumatism. Today's GPs might recognize that almost all these illnesses have now been eliminated or are eminently treatable.

By 1914, fever hospitals – hospitals that treated infectious diseases – were the largest single type of healthcare institution in England and Wales, with a total of over 31,000 beds, while rural hospitals specialized in conditions like tuberculosis. But as the management of fevers and infections came under control – at least in affluent countries – with public health measures, vaccination and eventually antibiotics, the focus of healthcare gradually shifted. The recent Covid-19 pandemic has emphasized just how far we had moved away from being ready to deal with large numbers of patients with infectious disease.

In the second half of the twentieth century, the primary paradigm of healthcare was relatively straightforward, at least from a medical perspective: acute medicine ruled. This was – and indeed it often still is – an era in which care was led by the specialist and the super-specialist. Medicine was subdivided into distinct medical specialties, conveniently dividing care needs into distinct packages. It was as if the medical establishment thought of patients as generally being well until they became sick – typically with a single condition – followed by death or recovery, with those who survived returning to normal life. Of course, there have always been chronic conditions, but during this era these rarely appeared to be the priority, and the planning of healthcare tended to focus on single illnesses.

The planning of hospitals focused on increasingly specialized departments – respiratory, cardiovascular, neurological, psychiatric and so on. Most medical education and research focused on these single areas, dealing with them one at a time. Medicine was designed around specialties and expertise, rather than necessarily around the overall needs of real patients. Nevertheless, dramatic improvements were made in the care of single conditions, with knowledge expanding exponentially.

In this medical world where the specialist was at the top of the tree, the generalist doctor was regarded as an anachronism. Specialism ruled, and doctors who had the smallest clinical focus – single conditions, or even parts of single conditions or of single organs – had the highest prestige. The generalists – particularly general practitioners and geriatricians – were frequently seen as a lesser clinical life form. In 1912, Sir Clifford Allbutt wrote a letter to *The Times* dismissing general practice as 'perfunctory work by perfunctory men'. And in 1949, Lord Moran, Winston Churchill's personal physician, said while giving evidence to a parliamentary committee that GPs 'have fallen from the ladder of advancement'. It is telling that each of these men was at one point president of the Royal College of Physicians.

Quite why a doctor who has to deal with everything is seen as having lower prestige than a doctor who deals with one very small area of care has always been a mystery to me. Returning to Sir James Mackenzie, his biographer wrote that choosing to become a family doctor 'meant that all hope of shining in his profession had been abandoned. Mackenzie knew very well that general practitioners do not shine. They are the rank and file, the common soldiers of the army of healing.' It was only when he began to focus on cardiology that his prestige and fame grew.

Attitudes like this persist to this day. Nearly a hundred years later, after a brief spell in hospital with a broken arm, my then six-year-old grandson described his mother as 'not being a proper doctor. She's just a GP.' It's fair to say that he and I had words!

This is illustrative of the pervasive nature of our focus on specialized care – single conditions and organs rather than whole humans. It is a paradigm that has delivered a great deal, but it is no longer always appropriate.

Over the last few decades, as a combination of improved healthcare and affluence have had a joint impact, much of healthcare has shifted away from treating acute illness to treating long-term problems. While phrases like 'the ageing population' or 'demographic change' are typically used to indicate a particular challenge or crisis, they actually signify astonishing success. It hardly needs saying, but the world's population is ageing because we aren't dying at as young an age. Media headlines continue to present this development in negative terms, but it's a remarkable and unprecedented success – a success that has come at a price.

As an example of how care has changed, consider our successes in the prevention and management of coronary artery disease, and particularly heart attacks. The changes in the past few decades have been truly astonishing and demonstrate how the challenges facing healthcare have dramatically changed.

In 1961, approximately 166,000 people died from coronary heart disease in Great Britain. In 2009, just forty-eight years later and despite the country having a significantly larger population, the number of deaths had more than halved, to around 80,000. Back in 1961, cardiovascular disease accounted for more than 50 per cent of all deaths in the UK, but by 2009 it had fallen to around a third,[20] a remarkable improvement.

In the US, a 2017 report from the American Heart Association showed that although it remains the leading cause of death in the US, deaths due to coronary heart disease have continued to decline over the past ten years.[21] However, the rate of decline has varied significantly in different communities. In another American study, researchers used data on heart disease deaths among people aged thirty-five and over between 1973 and 2010, finding that every single one of more than 3,000 counties saw a decline. However, there was a remarkable amount of variation. While the average decline across the US was 61 per cent, some counties only saw a decline of just 9 per cent, while others managed to cut their deaths by a remarkable 83 per cent.[22]

These huge variations are typically linked with affluence and poverty. Poor areas often have the poorest care and the poorest outcomes. It has long been the case that those with the greatest need tend to receive the least attention – a phenomenon described in 1971 by the Welsh family doctor Julian Tudor Hart as 'the inverse care law':

> The availability of good medical care tends to vary inversely with the need for it in the population served. This ... operates more completely where medical care is most exposed to market forces, and less so where such exposure is reduced.[23]

Tudor Hart would paraphrase his argument: 'To the extent that healthcare becomes a commodity it becomes distributed just like champagne. That is, rich people gets lots of it. Poor people don't get any of it.' He later regretted having coined a term that had entered the vocabulary of healthcare policy without leading to effective action. As Professor Graham Watt of Glasgow University has pointed out:

> The inverse care law is not a law, but the consequence of policies that restrict needs-based care in communities with the poorest health. Noisier, more assertive and more powerful interests hold sway. There is a disconnect between the rhetoric of addressing health inequalities and the reality of healthcare where it is needed most.[24]

This variability also applies to nations. Across the world, the improvement in heart disease is most clearly seen in high-income countries, with poorer countries lagging behind.

Moreover, when you don't die of one condition, you have a greater chance of developing another. Doom-laden newspaper headlines about increasing cancer rates might equally be written as a celebration of falling heart disease rates. Inevitably, as cardiovascular disease has diminished, cancer has become more common. The increasing number of cases, or indeed of dementia patients, is reasonably seen as a worrying challenge, but it is to a certain extent the inevitable result of success. As we win one battle, we immediately face another – and the multiplicity of diseases all seem to have an infinite supply of reinforcements.

My father didn't have time to develop cancer – he died of a heart attack before he reached the age that I am now. Indeed, had I died at the same age as him, I would not have developed the cancer that I have recently undergone extensive and expensive treatment for. The fact that I required cancer treatment could be seen as an unintended consequence of my avoiding heart disease.

Of course, it is likely that my father would never have had his initial heart attack today. I am sure someone would have challenged him about his smoking habit and his weight. Even though he was a doctor himself, I can hardly ever remember him without a pipe in his hand, either smoking or endlessly tinkering with it, but we now understand the risks he was taking. The drugs he took for his high blood pressure were state of the art at the time, but they have now been almost abandoned. We realize that they had serious side effects, including cognitive impairment, constipation and debilitating depression, while offering little benefit.

Even if preventive measures hadn't worked, the acute treatment of heart attacks has improved immeasurably since my father's time. Dad died in 1964. In the 1960s and 1970s, treatments such as bypass surgery and percutaneous balloon angioplasty were pioneered, and the 1980s saw the development of stents, small devices that prop open a narrowed artery. If he had suffered his heart attack today, the outcome would almost certainly have been better. As a paper in *The Lancet* stated:

> Something profound happened to deaths from coronary heart disease after they peaked in 1968. Over a few decades, the age-adjusted coronary heart disease mortality rate gradually fell by half across much of the world ... Equally impressive – but less publicized – is the mechanism of this decline. Using a validated mortality model, a team led by the University of Liverpool in

the UK found roughly equal contributions from acute lifesaving treatments, better control of blood pressure, a reduction in smoking, the use of bypass surgery and angioplasty, better post-infarction care and increased physical activity. There was no single breakthrough, but a varied array of changes in many areas of prevention and treatment for cardiovascular disease.[25]

I'm very grateful to have avoided the heart disease that killed my dad, but it is important to accept that one phenomenal success in healthcare provision has led to an epidemic of other problems. The reduction of deaths from heart disease in such a short period of time is a wonderful achievement, but every time we don't die of one condition, we have a chance to develop another. That's life – in every sense. We all die of something, and that something is likely to need treatment or care.

Indeed, as Benjamin Franklin wrote back in 1789, 'in this world nothing can be said to be certain, except death and taxes', and those two eternal verities will come together repeatedly in this book. Indeed, *Death and Taxes* might have served as a good alternative title, but they are hardly words that cheer anyone up – other than undertakers and the taxman.

Age and ageing
As we learned earlier in the chapter, life expectancy has, at least until very recently, been increasing at a quite extraordinary rate. One might think that it will inevitably reach a limit, but it is hard to tell. Professor Tom Kirkwood, a world-renowned expert on the biology of ageing, has rejected the notion that humans are 'programmed' to die, saying there is no evidence of this in evolutionary biology.[26]

We know that cells have the capacity to repair themselves, but this is damaged through illness, poor nutrition or accidents, and eventually their ability to self-repair is impaired, which causes us to age.

Today, large numbers of people are entering old age with far less cellular damage than their parents and grandparents, which has extended lifespans and made healthy lives at older ages possible. How far this change might continue is impossible to answer, but Dr Elizabeth Blackburn, the former president of the Salk Institute for Biological Studies in California and a Nobel laureate for research into the genetics of ageing, believes that children born today have a chance of living to 150, and lifespans of 120 years may well soon be the norm. She has been quoted as saying that many of the diseases of old age that were previously regarded as inevitable may not be after all. It's entirely possible that life expectancy, for the affluent at least, will continue to improve. And as we have already learned, the longer you live, the greater your opportunity for developing new medical conditions.

Remember my description of the way hospital services have typically been designed around specialized departments? This model assumes that patients have one single condition, but while this was once appropriate, it is no longer the case. Today, the focus of much of Western medicine on individual diseases means that we risk seeing patients as a set of faulty parts that can be fixed in isolation, rather than aiming to balance the complex interactions of their possible multiple conditions.

Put yourself in the shoes of a former patient of mine whom I will call Harold. I was his family doctor for nearly three decades, and towards the end of his life I noted that he had developed coronary artery disease, hypertension, hyperlipidaemia, chronic kidney disease, diabetes, macular degeneration, osteoarthritis of the hip, prostate cancer and – perhaps unsurprisingly – depression. Almost every family doctor knows someone like Harold, with a similar collection of conditions.

Multimorbidity – the coexistence of two or more long-term medical conditions or diseases – is an increasingly important problem in healthcare systems around the world.[27] Although much of healthcare is still currently designed around single specialties, more patients in the UK have two or more long-term health problems than have one single problem.[28] Across the European Union, there are at least 50 million people with multimorbidity. And in some low- and middle-income countries, healthcare systems are facing the double whammy of an increase in long-term conditions and non-communicable diseases at the same time as epidemics of infectious disease such as HIV and TB.

This increase in multimorbidity isn't simply a result of the 'ageing population', even though the prevalence of long-term conditions does rise with age. Studies in Scotland have shown that there are more people with long-term conditions under the age of sixty-five than in the older age group, although this is largely because the population as a whole at this age is bigger.[29] Another study in Canada showed that the largest proportion of patients with multimorbidity were aged under sixty-five, stating that these patients have combinations of chronic conditions that require carefully tailored treatment.[30]

The majority of people aged over sixty-five have two or more long-term conditions; the majority of over seventy-fives have three or more; overall, the number of people with multiple conditions is rising. Although I'm pretty healthy, I have a couple of these conditions myself – not surprising given my age. However, there is a significant correlation with social deprivation, with the onset of multimorbidity occurring ten to fifteen years earlier among those living in deprived areas compared with those in more affluent areas.

Faced with these issues, in 2012 the Royal College of Physicians established the Future Hospital Commission to address concerns about the standards of care in hospitals and to make recommendations for providing patients with the safe, high-quality, sustainable care that they deserve.[31]

Quoting a patient who said, 'I don't want to be passed round the wards: I'm a person, not a parcel,' the report called for a return to generalism:

> Embedded within our recommendations is the need for a resurgence of general medicine. Specialists, of course, play an essential role in the acute hospital but we need to ensure that, in the future, specialists all possess expertise in general medicine as well as in their specialty; and that they are able to provide patients with the broad range of clinical skills that the majority of them so desperately need.

This focus on the individual human being may ultimately have a profound impact on affordability. Inevitably, subdividing the patient into different bits – each requiring different expertise, inputs, appointments and teams – may not necessarily be the most cost-effective way of delivering care.

Thankfully, in the UK, the vital importance of this challenge to the way healthcare has developed has been recognized. In a 2020 report looking at the future needs of medical education, Health Education England referred to 'a collective challenge to make a fundamental shift in medical education from a system that places disproportionate value on specialism to one that recognizes crucial value in a generalist training'.[32]

The conundrum, however, is whether a return to generalism can deliver the immensely complex treatments that our patients deserve. After all, scientific advance is telling us more and more about each condition, subdividing seemingly common problems into a multiplicity of rarer ailments. All the evidence suggests that the expertise offered by super-specialization will be required to deliver the most effective therapies, but to focus on this alone is to deny the complex reality of patients' lives.

How much is enough?

The affordability of healthcare has been a challenge for every generation. As far back as 1949, Aneurin Bevan, the father of the UK National Health Service, told the Labour Party Conference that 'it is the same story ... in every social service. There is greater demand ... because the standards of the working-class population are higher than ever they were before.'

Richard Crossman, a distinguished British minister of social services, was quoted as saying that it was inevitable that choices had to be made, and that it was delusional to believe that a growing economy would allow a nation to afford everything. He believed that demography, technology and rising expectations would 'always together be sufficient to make the standard of social services regarded as essential to a civilized community far more expensive than that community can afford'.[33]

These problems are not unique to the UK and the British National Health Service. For instance, in the US, healthcare costs have risen at an extraordinary rate. In 1960, they were $27.2 billion, 5 per cent of GDP. By 2016, they had reached $3.3 trillion, a remarkable 17.9 per cent of GDP.[34] In the UK, the trend has been similar. Total per capita health expenditure rose from £1,879 in 2011–12 to £2,106 in 2015–16.[35] This equates to a daily healthcare cost of £5.76 per man, woman and child in England.

Here are a few more examples of increasing healthcare spending, as a proportion of countries' GDP.[36]

Australia: 1970: 4.1 per cent   2008: 8.5 per cent
Canada: 1970: 6.9 per cent   2008: 10.4 per cent
Norway: 1970: 4.4 per cent   2008: 8.5 per cent

The alternative way of looking at this expenditure is per capita and adjusted for inflation. The comparisons are quite dramatic:

Australia: 1970: $236   2008: $3,353
Canada: 1970: $294   2008: $4,079
UK: 1970: $159   2008: $3,129
US: 1970 $356   2008: $7,538
Norway: 1970: $143   2008: $5,003

If these increases continue into the future, there will clearly come a point when the trajectory becomes unsustainable. During the modern era of healthcare, the delivery of care has evolved constantly. Parallel to this evolution, costs have escalated, expectations have changed, opportunities have arisen, advances have been made, and yet – because of these changes – funding has remained as challenging as ever. The population is living longer and generally healthier lives than ever, but the costs have spiralled. The better things get, the more expensive care seems to become; the funding challenge for healthcare has become increasingly clear.

A 2008 World Health Organization report made a valid point about the tendency of healthcare to focus on single issues, rather than being clear about how to maximize benefit for their populations:

> Global and, increasingly, national policy formulation processes have focused on single issues … while scant attention is given to the underlying constraints that hold up health systems' development in national contexts. Rather than improving their response capacity and anticipating new challenges, health systems seem to be drifting from one short-term priority to another, increasingly fragmented and without a clear sense of direction.[37]

This inability to focus on what matters is of fundamental importance. The report continued:

> it is clear that left to their own devices, health systems do not gravitate naturally towards the goals of health for all through primary healthcare as articulated in the Declaration of Alma-Ata.

Alma-Ata in Kazakhstan was the setting for a conference in 1978 that expressed the urgent need for action by governments, health and development workers and the world community to promote the health of all people, and which identified primary healthcare as key to the attainment of the goal.

The report went on, 'Health systems are developing in directions that contribute little to equity and social justice and fail to get the best health outcomes for their money.' The result of this failure to focus has resulted in a number of worrying trends: systems that disproportionately focus on a narrow offer of specialized curative care, where a focus on short-term results fragments service delivery and where a hands-off approach to governance has allowed the unregulated commercialization of health to flourish.

When addressing these challenges, governments have tended to use politics to determine their approach to budgeting. In democracies, they make a judgement about what matters most to voters. For instance, it has long been recognized that in a publicly funded healthcare system, it is almost impossible to deliver all three of quality, affordability and access; determining which of these three things is most important has a profound effect on prioritization.

For instance, the issue of access to general practitioners has often been politically challenging – quite reasonably, people hate having to wait for an appointment. In dealing with this issue, which has been politically controversial in a number of British general elections, a choice to prioritize two out of affordability, quality and access generally has to be made.

If the system prioritizes access and affordability, this is likely to mean compromising on quality. Alternatively, priority could be given to rapid access and quality, achieved by having more clinicians available to see patients, which would have a profound impact on affordability. Or the choice could be for quality and affordability, achieved by making people wait to be seen. This has traditionally been the model that has evolved in many healthcare systems. You can have good care, but you have to wait for it.

The only alternative solution to this dilemma is by innovating, choosing to do things differently and being clear about a healthcare system's limitations and boundaries. The coronavirus pandemic resulted in a much-increased use of virtual consultations. At the time of writing, it is too early to judge what the impact of this will be on patient satisfaction and outcomes, though research will certainly focus on the potential benefits and unintended consequences. While many patients value the option of virtual or online consultations, others – particularly some older citizens – feel they are being deprived if they do not have a face-to-face in-person consultation with a doctor on every occasion, a line that has been taken by a number of mass-market newspapers. With current workforce shortages and levels of demand, this is unlikely to be a practical option in the future, but ways of minimizing any digital divide will be critically important.

To make life even more complex, there is increasing evidence that continuity of care with a general practitioner really matters. A research paper from Norway in 2021 showed that patients who stayed registered with the same GP over many years had fewer out-of-hours appointments and acute hospital admissions, as well as a reduced risk of death.[38]

These benefits were significant, and they increased the longer the relationship continued. In 2018, people who had kept the same GP for more than fifteen years had a 25 per cent lower chance of dying than those with a GP relationship lasting a year or less. These are astonishing benefits, but it should be noted that Norwegian general practitioners care for half the number of patients as their UK equivalents. If drugs produced benefits of this scale, massive investment would be found to provide them. Instead, British governments repeatedly prioritize rapid access over continuity. After all, access problems cause headlines. Continuity problems tend to be invisible, although many older people privately mourn the passing of the phrase 'my doctor'.

Meanwhile, costs continue to rise, and there is no reason to think this might end any time soon. There is always more that can be done, more that *might* be paid for and more that patients will say 'should' be paid for. In the UK, although Aneurin Bevan recognized the potential impact of this ever-increasing cost, he stated that 'Illness is neither an indulgence for which people have to pay, nor an offence for which they should be penalized, but a misfortune, the cost of which should be shared by the community.'

Other countries chose to take a different path, but one simple fact remained. However healthcare might be funded, there will never be enough money to pay for everything – so tough decisions have to be made. The key question is, how?

CHAPTER 3

Paying the Price

Imagine that a brand-new country has come into being. Perhaps a massive volcanic eruption has formed a new island similar to Surtsey, which appeared off the southern coast of Iceland in 1963. Our theoretical island – let's call it Isla Santé – is far enough away from any other state to avoid being annexed to their political infrastructure. It is large, stable and attractive, with sufficient natural resources to make it wealthy enough to rapidly develop a sizeable and significant population.

However much the government of Isla Santé may concentrate on doing everything that they can to design policies to address poverty, loneliness, under-education, malnutrition and the many other social determinants of ill health, their citizens will inevitably become ill or need care. It may be something as simple as a broken arm, or it may be as complex as an acute and aggressive leukaemia. If we assume that the island's location makes outsourcing the care of its population to another state either impossible or impractical, it will need doctors, nurses, healthcare facilities and all the clinical and non-clinical staff required to run a safe and effective health service – physiotherapists, porters, educators, therapists, dieticians, radiographers, managers, planners, pharmacists and so on.

These professionals, buildings and equipment don't come cheap – even if we ignore the cost of training them to a safe and competent level. For instance, if you try to source an MRI scanner online, you'll find yourself reading blog posts like this:

> How much does an MRI machine cost? MRI systems are found within the wide price range of 30,000 to 700,000 euros ... It is often the finances that set the limit to which MRI system you can purchase, but the first thing to do is to identify your needs.[1]

You may find it jarring to read such advertisements, but it is important to remember that healthcare is a business. Once you have your equipment, running costs can also be remarkably high. Operating theatres, for instance, are one of the most expensive areas in a hospital to run, with an average cost of approximately £1,200 per hour.[2]

Inevitably, these costs vary quite remarkably from nation to nation. Let's take the example of a hip prosthesis, the artificial joint that so many people (including me) have had inserted to free them from pain and disability. There are a wide range of different prostheses that surgeons can choose to use, and they vary greatly in price depending on the design. The average price paid in different countries varies widely, too.[3]

As an example, the average cost of a hip prosthesis in 2013 was $3,177 in Spain, $6,723 in New Zealand, $9,982 in Australia and $11,806 in the US. I'll leave you to ponder why those prices might be so very different, though it may not take you too long.

Incidentally, a hip prosthesis is not an outlier – I've chosen it because it provides a typical example of the international variability in the expense of medical equipment. A recent report by the International Federation of Health Plans quoted various international prices for many other medical procedures.[4] For a typical angioplasty, a procedure that opens a blocked blood vessel to the heart, the average price in the US is $32,200, compared with $6,400 in the Netherlands and $7,400 in Switzerland. An MRI scan typically costs $1,420 in the United States but around $450 in Britain. An injection of Herceptin, a breast cancer treatment, costs $211 in the United States, compared with $44 in South Africa.

However you might choose to look at it, these wonderful innovations are extremely expensive. Healthcare systems use hip replacement prostheses by the thousand, and their cost does not include the cost of the operating theatre, the nurses, the anaesthetist, the drugs, the physiotherapy, the meals in hospital while you recover from the operation, the wages of the porter who takes you to and from the theatre, the bandages, the stitches, the mop that is used to clean the floor of the ward, the lightbulbs in the corridors, the crutches you use on the way home, the electricity that powers the hospital, the daily living aids you use when you get home and anything else that will be required. This is why if you pay for it yourself, the average cost of a total hip replacement in the UK is currently more than £10,000, based on the price lists of 175 private hospitals. When I Googled the question 'How much is a hip replacement?', the lowest quoted price was £7,600, the highest was £16,764 and the median was £10,761.

In the US, patients without health insurance who require a total hip replacement have to pay between $31,839 and $44,816, with an average cost of $39,299, according to Blue Cross Blue Shield of North Carolina.[5] And in Australia, the cost of hip replacement surgery ranges from $22,000 to $25,000, with approximately $800 incurred as additional out-of-pocket costs, as well as further associated costs after the surgery in the form of radiographic check-ups.[6] The cost will inevitably vary in other countries, but it is unlikely to be cheap – wherever you live, healthcare is an expensive business.

In the last chapter I mentioned the 'inverse care law', which states that people who need the best care tend to get the worst, and vice versa. This applies as much to nations as much as it does within populations. A 2008 report by the World Health Organization looking at the pattern of healthcare delivery around the world[7] identified some common contradictions. It turns out that those people with the greatest means – and whose need for healthcare is often less – consume the most care, whereas those with the least means – and the greatest problems – consume the least. In high- and low-income countries alike, public spending on health services most often benefits the rich more than the poor.

The report also showed that where people lack social protection and payment for care largely comes out of their own pocket, they can be confronted with massive and catastrophic expenses. Around the world, over 100 million people fall into poverty every year as a result of healthcare expenses. But as the report said, 'In modern states, governments are expected to protect health, to guarantee access to healthcare and to safeguard people from the impoverishment that illness can bring.' It is clear that many governments are letting their populations down.

Different nations, different approaches
Before we look at the challenge of controlling escalating costs, this chapter will look at the ways in which different nations have dealt with the problem facing the government of our mythical island of Isla Santé. They may tackle the problem in different ways, but the real issue is the same: healthcare costs real money, which someone has to pay – and no amount of wishful thinking can avoid this

simple fact. Some countries have made this issue the responsibility of the individual citizen, while others put most of the responsibility onto the state. No one has a perfect system, and there are benefits and risks to each approach.

In recent years, the World Health Organization and the United Nations have each expressed a clear and noble ambition for global healthcare, with 'universal health coverage' (UHC) being the primary aspiration. A country that offers it is defined as having citizens who can access health services without incurring financial hardship.[8] Dr Margaret Chan, a former director general of the WHO, has described UHC as the 'single most powerful concept that public health has to offer', since it unifies 'services and delivers them in a comprehensive and integrated way'.[9]

The member states of the United Nations have agreed to work towards worldwide universal health coverage by 2030.[10] However, this does not mean that citizens should have unlimited coverage for anything and everything. According to the WHO, UHC means that all individuals and communities receive the health services they need – including the full spectrum of essential services, from health promotion to prevention, treatment, rehabilitation and palliative care – without suffering financial hardship.

UHC enables every citizen to access the services that address the most important causes of disease and death, while ensuring that their quality is good enough to improve the health of the people who receive them. It is designed to protect people from the financial consequences of paying for health services out of their own pockets, which significantly 'reduces the risk that people will be pushed into poverty because unexpected illness requires them to use up their life savings, sell assets, or borrow – destroying their futures and often those of their children'.[11]

In 2015, when the UN introduced their Sustainable Development Goals, achieving UHC was one of the most critical. The WHO has noted that progression towards this goal will enable progress towards other health-related targets – good health allows children to learn and adults to earn, helping people escape poverty while providing the basis for long-term economic development.

The WHO has also made a number of important observations regarding what UHC is *not* designed to achieve. For instance, it does not mean free coverage for *all* possible health interventions, as no country can sustainably provide all services free of charge. According to the WHO, UHC is about not only ensuring a minimum package of health services but ensuring an expansion of services and financial protection as resources become available. It is not simply about individual treatment services but also includes population-based services such as public health campaigns and the addition of fluoride to water.

Universal health coverage is a noble aspiration that Dr Tedros Adhanom Ghebreyesus, the WHO director general, summarized in 2018. He said: 'Universal health coverage is a political choice. It takes vision, courage and long-term thinking. But the payoff is a safer, fairer and healthier world for everyone.'[12] He added, 'When you are building a house, you can't start to construct the walls before you have laid the foundations. Ensuring that everyone can access affordable healthcare, right in the heart of their communities, is the foundation for everything else we are trying to achieve.' He also made it clear that primary healthcare must be the bedrock of UHC, with an emphasis on promoting health and preventing disease. Amen to that.

However noble the aspiration, the fact remains that health services have to be paid for – although studies have shown that greater spending does not always lead to better outcomes. Japan's universal health coverage is a good example to those aspiring to achieve UHC at a relatively low cost, having been recognized internationally for its achievements during the second half of the twentieth century in improving the population's health and developing a strong healthcare system.[13] Nevertheless, as the WHO has stated, 'No country has made significant progress towards universal health coverage without increasing the extent to which its health system relies on public revenue sources.'

For most states with UHC, revenue from general taxation is the main source of funding, but this can be supplemented by specific levies that are paid either by individuals or employers. In addition, some services are not covered by the publicly funded system; these need to be paid for either directly or by insurance.

The world's first social health insurance system was almost certainly introduced in Germany. Bismarck's Health Insurance Act of 1883 was built on the same principles of solidarity and self-governance that have remained at the core of its development ever since.[14] In Europe, most healthcare systems are funded by a mix of public and private payment. Healthcare in Sweden, Denmark, Spain and Portugal is primarily funded by tax revenue, while Germany and France fund it through private and public contributions. Of course, we should be aware that whether money is found through taxation or comes directly from patients' pockets, it is the *same money*. When politicians vow to reduce taxation, they seem to ignore the fact that the cost of care will still need to be paid for somehow.

In the UK, the National Health Service is funded almost entirely through taxation. While the service is regarded by many as a world-leading system in state-provided healthcare, it isn't always viewed so positively outside the UK. I recall being asked repeatedly while working as a medical student in Providence, Rhode Island in 1970 what I felt about working in a system of socialized medicine, with the clear implication from many of my colleagues that it was akin to a form of communism. The reaction to recent healthcare reform in the US suggests that this attitude still exists. As one American author has written, 'The claim that there is a "right to healthcare" violates the principle of individual rights because it requires that the liberty of doctors and the property of taxpayers be violated to provide for others.'[15] I guess we will all respond rather differently to a sentence like that.

It was the German insurance system that stimulated a change to healthcare funding in the UK. After visiting Germany in 1908, the British chancellor David Lloyd George announced in his next Budget speech that Britain should aim to be 'putting ourselves in this field on a level with Germany'. As a result, the 1911 National Insurance Act provided healthcare coverage for those in work, initially through family doctors rather than hospitals. The main driver for this initiative was concern about poverty – Lloyd George was keen that the state should help those who became poor through ill health.

The insurance scheme allowed employer, employee and the state to contribute to a fund when the worker was employed, so that if the worker became ill, they could receive money for a limited period of time. Insured workers were entitled to ten shillings (50p in modern currency) per week for thirteen weeks and five shillings (25p) for another thirteen weeks if they were ill. After twenty-six weeks of sickness, workers were on their own and had to rely on Poor Law medical facilities.

In addition, workers were entitled to free medical treatment and thirty shillings in maternity benefit for the birth of each child. However, it was only the workers themselves who received benefits

– their families weren't covered, and nor were the self-employed and the unemployed. The healthcare aspects of this initial act were focused on addressing one potential cause of poverty in the workforce, and it continued through to the Second World War.

Many people, of course, were left without cover, and the vast number of casualties during the Second World War reduced the healthcare system to near bankruptcy. At the time, the UK's 2,700 hospitals were run by either councils or charities. The only people entitled to free treatment were those with jobs, but the massive impact of war combined with prior under-investment had reduced the system to a desperate state.

Action was needed, so in 1948 the provision of medical care became free and based on need rather than the ability to pay. The NHS was financed through taxation, with the rich contributing more than the poor. It was an extraordinary development.

According to the NHS historian Geoffrey Rivett:

> The history of the NHS is that of an organization established after a century's discussion on the provision of health services to meet a long-recognized need ... The cataclysm of war provided an opportunity that might not have been taken in quieter times ... Whether knowing what we know now Britain would follow the same pathway towards a universal healthcare system is anyone's guess.[16]

The birth of the NHS

To my mind, the creation of the NHS was one of humankind's most noble undertakings. At its birth, a leaflet was sent to every household in the UK, promising that the NHS 'will provide you with all medical, dental and nursing care. Everyone – rich or poor – can use it. There are no charges, except for a few special items. There are no insurance qualifications. But it is not a "charity". You are all paying for it, mainly as taxpayers, and it will relieve your money worries in time of illness.'

Whatever your view of the NHS, what happened next was key. Demand for healthcare almost immediately exceeded all predictions, with the number of patients on doctors' registers rising to 30 million. The NHS had budgeted £1 million for opticians, but within a year it had issued 5.25 million spectacle prescriptions. In 1947, doctors were issuing 7 million prescriptions per month; by 1951, this number had risen to 19 million per month.[17]

For the first time, many of the poorest people in society gained access to doctors and treatments that had previously been beyond their means. However, what followed was one of the great miscalculations in the history of healthcare. It was assumed that after an initial surge in demand, the cost of the service would fall as the backlog of needs was dealt with. People would be healthier and would need less care as a result. This theory seemed perfectly logical, but it could not have been further from reality. The initial estimate was that the NHS would cost £132 million each year; in its first year of operation, it spent over £300 million. The challenge of spiralling healthcare cost is not a new one.

In June 1948, the month before the NHS was founded, Aneurin Bevan addressed a Royal College of Nursing conference. 'We shall never have all we need,' he said. 'Expectations will always exceed capacity. The service must always be changing, growing and improving – it must always appear inadequate.'[18]

In February 1953, the UK treasury requested an inquiry into the

NHS and related expenditure.[19] The report, published in 1956, far from finding any way to substantially reduce the annual cost of the service, stated that expenditure was too low and that the NHS's record 'was one of real achievement'.

As the costs of the service were so high, some charges had to be introduced. In 1952, prescription charges of one shilling (5p) and a flat rate of £1 for dental treatment were introduced. The prescription charges were abolished in 1965, before being reintroduced three years later. In England, while there are a large number of exemptions, these charges have persisted ever since. Indeed, in a recent year, over one billion prescriptions were issued. Although 89.4 per cent of them were issued free of charge and the income from fees makes up less than 1 per cent of the NHS budget, every little helps.

Costs have continued to spiral. In 1949–50, the UK health budget was £0.4 billion. In 2017, it was £197.4 billion. If this increase had been caused by inflation alone, the 2017 figure would have been £117 billion – a massive level of spending, but £80 billion less than the actual figure.

Before we leave the example of the UK, it is worth stressing that several specific societal factors applied when the NHS was established, many of which have since changed dramatically. In the late 1940s, the population trusted that the government could deliver. The country had just won the Second World War, a success that involved spectacular levels of centralized planning and delivery. Secondly, medical science at the time was relatively limited. Treatment was much cheaper, and therefore more affordable. The population also had much lower expectations of healthcare – a long way from today's assumption that there should be 'a pill for every ill'. We have shifted to a remarkable cultural reliance on medicine and medicines. In 1949, the British National Formulary contained around 250 drugs; today, it comprises over 18,000. Consulting rates have also escalated dramatically since 1948. These factors would likely have a massive impact if a similar system was introduced now.

I've so far focused on the UK, as it was one of the first countries – and certainly the most prominent – to provide genuine universal health coverage. But everywhere in the world has faced the same challenges – ever-increasing demand and costs, leading to a problem regarding how it should be funded.

The Second World War was a major influence in the establishment of healthcare systems around the world. New Zealand created a universal healthcare system between 1939 and 1941, while the Australian state of Queensland introduced a state-paid public hospital system in the 1940s. The UK system was established in 1948, followed by the Scandinavian countries – Sweden in 1955, Norway and Iceland in 1956, Denmark in 1961 and Finland in 1964. Japan introduced universal health coverage in 1961 and Canada introduced it province by province between 1962 and 1972, although Canadian Medicare for hospital care had been introduced in Saskatchewan in 1947.[20] Full universal health insurance was implemented across Australia with the Medibank system in 1975, which led to universal coverage under the Medicare system in 1984.

Between the 1970s and the early twenty-first century, many other European countries began to introduce universal health coverage, building upon pre-existing health insurance programmes. South Korea, Taiwan and Thailand came next, Russia built on its pre-existing system after the fall of the Soviet Union, and more recent years have seen the development of UHC in Latin America, much of Africa and the Caribbean. China has the most ambitious scheme of all. A few years ago, I was privileged to meet the Chinese vice-minister for health, who talked about the demands of providing care for 1.3 billion people – an eye-watering challenge.

With 195 countries in the world, it is impossible to describe every single variation that has evolved to address the challenge of how to fund healthcare. Nevertheless, most countries can be grouped into a series of approaches, ranging from tax-based funding (with or without user fees to top up payment) and single-payer healthcare to various types of insurance scheme.

In reality, most countries – particularly in Europe – use a range of different models, with taxation the most common source of funding. Sometimes the tax-funded benefits are restricted, with citizens having to pay for additional services – either directly or through an insurance scheme.

Some people argue that the whole concept of universal health coverage is an infringement of an individual's human rights. They say that those with money are transferring their wealth through taxation to pay for the healthcare of those who do not have money, and that everyone should instead be personally and exclusively responsible for themselves and their families.

Other people argue the exact opposite; that providing access to health for the whole population is hugely beneficial for society. After all, we share the cost of the military who risk their lives to protect us and the fire service who rescue us in times of peril – why should healthcare be less of a societal issue?

The fact that people have such different opinions about these fundamental issues makes the funding of healthcare uniquely political, with a tendency for debate to be more ideological than practical. I know where I stand – I agree with Mahatma Gandhi, who said, 'The true measure of any society can be found in how it treats its most vulnerable members.' You may think differently, but that doesn't take away from the fact that money is needed for healthcare, whoever pays for it.

The best system?
You might have thought that we would by now have some definitive evidence for which funding system delivers the best results. If only it was that simple. In fact, there is an extraordinary lack of correlation between what countries spend and the results they achieve – and this will be a recurring theme throughout this book. Comparing the Caribbean island of Cuba and the mighty United States illustrates the lack of correlation between healthcare expenditure and outcomes.

There are lessons to be learned from the contrasting approaches to healthcare funding of Cuba and the US. Cuba offers universal health coverage to its citizens, which costs about 7.6 per cent of its GDP. Its health indicators, which are known to be the best in Latin America, are better than those of the US in some important respects, including infant mortality rates, underweight babies, HIV infection, immunization rates and the per capita number of doctors. The US – which on these criteria gets worse results – spends 17.9 per cent of its GDP on health, a quite extraordinary difference.

In late August 2005, following the destruction of New Orleans by Hurricane Katrina, a highly symbolic story hit the headlines: the Cuban leader Fidel Castro contacted the Bush administration and offered to send 1,600 doctors and many tons of medical supplies to Louisiana's worst-affected areas.[21] The offer was refused – a sad outcome, but understandable from a political perspective. However, that doesn't mean that the US has nothing to learn from Cuba. In the Cuban province of Cienfuegos, just three babies per 1,000 die, while in the considerably wealthier United States, the data shows that there are nearly six deaths for every 1,000 live births.

Indeed, Cuba's infant mortality rates match those in Canada and the United Kingdom. There are massive societal differences between these countries, and the standard of living for most of the two populations is barely comparable. But when it comes to the provision of healthcare, money, it seems, is not everything.

Of course, if you are rich or adequately insured in the US, you are likely to receive the very best care in the world. But if you are poor, the results can be much worse than are achieved in Cuba. Many people feel that caring for all its citizens – and particularly those who are least able to care for themselves – is a key responsibility of any government, though the rights and wrongs of this debate belong in another book. The wrath that any mention of Obamacare seemed to trigger among some Americans suggests that the concept of universal health coverage in the US has some way to go. Nevertheless, a number of states, including Minnesota, Connecticut and Massachusetts, have taken serious steps towards universal healthcare, while Oregon and the city of San Francisco have governments that understand the value of universal healthcare.

Remember that the US spends 17.9 per cent of its GDP on healthcare, more than double the expenditure of any other country. Is this money spent well? Well, it has been shown that a randomly selected American aged between forty-five and fifty-four is more than twice as likely to die early as someone from the same age group in Sweden. For every 400 middle-aged Americans who die each year, 220 die in Australia, 230 in Britain, 290 in Germany and 300 in France.[22] Indeed, although it spends more on healthcare than any other nation, and despite the high quality of many American hospitals, the US is thirty-first in global rankings of life expectancy, behind countries like Cyprus and Chile. The shortfall in the quality of its care is partly driven by the extraordinary administrative costs.

While the US healthcare sector has about 800,000 practising physicians, nearly twice that number are employed to administer its payment system. In 2018, a *New York Times* report showed that out of the $19,000 that US workers, on average, paid each year for family healthcare coverage, about $5,700 went towards administrative costs.[23] Some years ago, the American journalist Walter Cronkite said that 'America's healthcare system is neither healthy, caring, nor a system' – and he was right.

It is ironic that while the US is the only OECD country without universal health coverage, it continues to lead the world in medical research. One such area of research is carried out by the Commonwealth Fund in Massachusetts, which presents an overview of healthcare systems around the world. The below chart shows that although the proportion of GDP spent by the US is double that of the UK, the US still manages to perform worst on almost every measurable criterion.

Healthcare System Performance Rankings (as reported by the Commonwealth Fund)[24]

	AUS	CAN	FRA	GER	NETH	NZ	NOR	SWE	SWIZ	UK	US
Overall Ranking	3	10	8	5	2	6	1	7	9	4	11
Access to Care	8	9	7	3	1	5	2	5	10	4	11
Care Process	6	4	10	9	3	1	8	11	7	5	2
Administrative Efficiency	2	7	6	9	8	3	1	5	10	4	11
Equity	1	10	7	2	5	9	8	6	3	4	11
Healthcare Outcomes	1	10	6	7	4	8	2	5	3	9	11

These international comparisons can be instructive. A different way of comparing countries is to look at the health costs per person, calculated in purchasing power parity (PPP), which aims to provide equivalence between countries – so that $1 spent in the US, for instance, goes as far as $1 spent in India. A major advantage of using PPP is that it is both a currency converter and a price deflator, so the results should theoretically reflect only the difference in the volumes of goods and services consumed in those countries.

Using PPP, it is possible to compare annual health expenditure per capita. The World Bank has published a chart on this,[25] and the differences are extraordinary. Let's look at a selection of nations in ascending order, using the data for 2016:

Democratic Republic of the Congo: $34
Afghanistan: $163
China: $762
Brazil: $1,777
Cyprus: $2,271
New Zealand: $3,665
United Kingdom: $4,178
Australia: $4,530
Canada: $4,718
France: $4,782
Netherlands: $5,251
Ireland: $5,300
Germany: $5,463
United States: $9,870

All the numbers may have caused your eyes to blur over, but the current health expenditure per capita in the US is double that of France and more than double that of the UK and Canada, and yet the US is bottom of the previous table for healthcare outcomes. If anything demonstrates that more money does not automatically buy you an increase in quality, it is this. But if every American citizen could experience the level of healthcare experienced by the most affluent, the cost would be beyond astronomical.

Another example of the lack of correlation between expenditure and results is Brazil, which is at the lower end of spending but has had remarkable results. Infant mortality has dropped from 48 per 1,000 to 17 per 1,000. In just the past five years, hospital admissions due to diabetes or stroke have decreased by 25 per cent, the proportion of children under five years old who are underweight has fallen by 67 per cent, over 75 per cent of women now receive seven or more antenatal consultations, and diphtheria, tetanus and pertussis (DTP) vaccine coverage in children less than one year old is greater than 95 per cent in most municipalities.[26]

An alternative way of looking at the differences between countries is to look at the average per capita healthcare spending using countries' internationally accepted economic descriptor bands.[27]

	Total government spending on healthcare (%)	Spending per person
Global	15.4	$863 PPP
Low-Income	8.7	$67 PPP
Lower-Middle-Income	7.8	$181 PPP
Upper-Middle-Income	9.4	$757 PPP
High-Income	17.2	$4,405 PPP

The most striking aspect of these comparisons is that the poorest countries are the ones in which healthcare costs are most often paid for by patients directly – even though their populations are least likely to be able to afford it. As a report from the World Health Organization stated:

> Treatment for diabetes, cancer, cardiovascular disease and chronic respiratory disease can be protracted and therefore extremely expensive. Such costs can force families into catastrophic spending and impoverishment … Each year, an estimated 100 million people are pushed into poverty because they have to pay directly for health services.[28]

This problem isn't going to ease any time soon. Indeed, every single graph indicates that costs are going up every year. But to complicate matters further, our aspirations are continuing to change.

Changing expectations
Different generations have wildly different expectations around healthcare – both in terms of what they will tolerate and their attitude to waiting or paying for care. In England, the older generation's view might be summed up by the phrase 'Mustn't grumble.' In my own rural practice, I recall meeting elderly farmers who would tolerate the most extraordinary disability, regarding it as something they expected to happen as they aged. Meanwhile, younger generations are often far less tolerant, expecting problems to be treated with much more urgency, with a general perception that there is a 'pill for every ill'. Neither outlook is right or wrong but they are very different, which has an inevitable impact on the demand for healthcare. The more that is seen as possible, the more it is expected, which is yet another driver towards increased cost.

When it comes to mental health issues, the problem is even more complex. The definition of what might be an acceptable level of stress to endure, for instance, has shifted from generation to generation. How can one possibly compare the stress of huddling in an air raid shelter after your home has been destroyed and members of your family have been killed with the stress of being bullied at work? And yet the latter can be so distressing that it leads to many suicides. According to the World Health Organization, nearly 800,000 people – one person every forty seconds – die due to suicide every year, and research indicates that for each adult who dies by suicide, more than twenty may attempt it.[29] As societies become more affluent, the pain that drives some people to suicide does not appear to be lessening. If mental health conditions were prioritized in the same way as cancer, every country would need to significantly increase its healthcare provision.

There is no definitive way of classifying depression, stress or anxiety that equates to the diagnostic appearance of a rash in measles or a mass in cancer, but that does not make these conditions less real – it simply means that what society and individuals will accept is shifting, and will continue to do so. In recent years, countless media interviews with people experiencing difficulties in life refer to their mental health, when in the past they might just have referred to feeling sad, distressed, worried, unhappy or anxious. It is wonderful that people feel more comfortable talking about their mental health than they might have done in the past – and I am in no way implying that their distress is anything other than very real – but when boundaries of health and disease are so flexible, determining the optimum level of provision – and therefore of the budget required – becomes increasingly and extraordinarily difficult. And these problems are not going to go away.

CHAPTER 4

Why Is it All So Expensive?

The chapters so far have highlighted the challenges and dilemmas that result from the ever-increasing cost of healthcare – an interesting contrast to the falling prices that we see in so many other aspects of life. While most tech equipment seems to plummet in price – even as its specifications improve – it is clear that for many healthcare technologies, diagnostics and drugs, the exact opposite seems to apply. Impressions can be misleading, but if this is true, what are the explanations? And what might be the solutions?

It's not just that the technologies get more expensive – the fact that we keep on moving the goal posts doesn't help. I have already mentioned the flawed assumption in Britain following the introduction of the NHS that a cared-for population would be healthier and would require less care. Instead, every time we solve one problem, we seem to create another. Do we know what the endgame is, or do we just keep on buying more of the expensive products because we feel it would be immoral to stop? And if we look at healthcare systems as a whole, can we be sure that we are investing our money in the most effective way?

This is why we need to talk about cost. Why it is so high, and what might the potential benefits and challenges of personalized medicine and genomics be?

The cost of anything has two main variables – the product and the customer's needs. This book has so far repeatedly alluded to the challenges of an ageing population. A combination of public health measures, educational improvements and effective medical care has led to a magnificent increase in life expectancy for people across the globe, an increase for which we should all be immensely grateful. But it is clear that ageing on its own does not directly increase healthcare costs. Instead, research has shown that multimorbidity – the increasing number of health conditions and age-related impairments – and proximity to death are more strongly linked to healthcare costs than age. A study in the UK investigating healthcare showed that costs in people over the age of eighty increased until they reached their mid-nineties, before declining again. Proximity to death was the strongest predictor of cost, which was highest for people aged between eighty and eighty-four: £10,027 per year, compared to £7,021 per year for those over one hundred. It is fairly obvious that if you live to the age of one hundred, you are likely to be pretty healthy. Where patients had multiple illnesses, that had a strong influence, with each additional health complaint increasing costs.[1]

In healthcare, the product is made up of many different factors – including staff, drugs, surgery and buildings, as well as the many different types of care that may be offered. For instance, a report from the UK's Office for National Statistics on the country's health expenditure for 2016 showed that 63.9 per cent of the healthcare budget was spent on curative and rehabilitation care, 15.5 per cent on long-term care, 10.5 per cent on medical goods and 5.1 per cent on prevention.[2] The total expenditure on healthcare in that year was £191.7 billion – another eye-watering figure that might be more meaningful when expressed as £191,700,000,000.

Where, and why, is all this money spent? In an industry where care is central, it is inevitable that the main cost is people. The NHS currently employs about 1.5 million people in England,[3] making it the world's fifth largest employer after the US Department of Defense, the Chinese army, Walmart and McDonald's.[4] The NHS is heavily reliant on qualified clinical staff, who account for around half of its employees. The vast majority of staff – 1.1 million full-time equivalents – work in 'hospital and community services' as direct employees of NHS trusts, where they provide ambulance, mental health, community and hospital services. In addition, around 130,000 people work in primary care.

Many people repeatedly express concern about the number of managers – a feeling that is fuelled by certain newspapers and politicians – but fewer than 3 per cent of NHS employees are managerial.[5] Indeed, the coronavirus pandemic has highlighted the vitally important role that managers play. After all, emergency hospitals, treatment centres, vaccination rollouts and services don't design and build themselves.

It is clear that the reasons that costs are so high, and increasing every year, are multifactorial, with doctors and hospitals being the prime driver. But the more you look into this issue, the less straightforward it is. In a powerful essay for the *New Yorker* in 2009, Atul Gawande – a surgeon, public health researcher and writer – examined the huge variability in cost between comparable American communities.[6] He noted that McAllen, a city in southern Texas with a population of around 150,000, was one of the most expensive healthcare markets in the country, with only Miami spending more per person. Gawande wrote:

> In 2006, Medicare spent fifteen thousand dollars per enrolee here, almost twice the national average. The income per capita is twelve thousand dollars. In other words,

> Medicare spends three thousand dollars more per person here than the average person earns [...] McAllen costs Medicare seven thousand dollars more per person each year than does the average city in America. But not, so far as one can tell, because it's delivering better healthcare.

Gawande's conclusion was stark. The primary cause of McAllen's extreme costs, he realized, was the overuse of medicine – procedures that simply didn't need to be done. In healthcare, doing more is not always better. We expect doctors only to do those things that are necessary. While there may be unethical individuals who maximize their income by carrying out profitable procedures unnecessarily, much of this over-activity has simply become normal practice. Operations are done because they have always been done, leading clinicians to continue making the same mistakes with ever-increasing confidence.

Take the example of arthroscopy, a type of keyhole surgery that involves washing out the knee joint to treat osteoarthritis. In many countries around the world the procedure became extremely common, but in 2007, the UK National Institute for Health and Care Excellence examined the evidence of its benefits and concluded that such treatments should not be offered for osteoarthritis, unless the patient has knee osteoarthritis with a clear history of 'mechanical locking'. Nevertheless, ten years later, more than 2 million of these procedures were still being performed worldwide each year, at an annual cost of $3 billion in the US alone.[7]

Too much medicine
Why do clinicians persist in carrying out such low-benefit procedures? After all, where healthcare systems have finite budgets, carrying out an unnecessary and expensive procedure on patient A

might limit the funds that are available for a proven and effective procedure on patient B. A paper in 'Health Policy' looked at the biases that can come into play when a clinician fails to follow the best guidance around prioritizing care.[8] For instance, the patient who is sitting in front of the clinician will inevitably take priority over those who are not, which means that resources tend to be based more on patient demand than on justice or equity. It is only natural that when we consult doctors, we want them to be focused on us alone. But when we are citizens or taxpayers, we want them to think of society.

Other biases the paper flagged up included 'failure embarrassment effect' – it is natural to be disinclined to admit that a treatment we have been offering for years is of low or no benefit – and the 'status quo effect', which leads us to prefer what is known and comfortable. 'Risk aversion' is another powerful bias. In a complex, expensive and challenging medico-legal world, clinicians often feel that it is better to be criticized for doing something than for *not* doing something, which leads them to practise what is described as 'defensive medicine'.

In this paper, two further examples of biases struck me as particularly relevant. 'Availability heuristics' is a bias by which something is used because it is there rather than because of any distinct clinical need – the idea of 'scan because you can'. I have always taught (and tried to practise) the importance of only carrying out an investigation if you have an idea what you might do with the result. If all you do is file it away, why did you carry out the investigation in the first place? Would a different result really have changed your plans? The final bias is the 'boys and toys effect'. Technology may be fun and interesting, but its use may come at an opportunity cost for other patients.[9]

WHY IS IT ALL SO EXPENSIVE?

The factors that influence clinical decisions are clearly less straightforward than we might think. I know I've been guilty on many occasions of thinking that doing more must be preferable to doing less – there are some situations when you feel that 'something must be done'. But the best advice, it turns out, is often that given by the White Rabbit to Alice in Walt Disney's *Alice in Wonderland*: 'Don't just do something. Stand there!'

Finally, politicians and journalists are often coerced by pressure groups who push for the availability of expensive facilities to treat their particular condition. Lobbying can make a major impact, but such decisions should be based on rational evidence rather than emotive arguments, particularly when the lobbyist is funded by the equipment's manufacturers. Evidence matters.

A number of healthcare systems around the world are beginning to tackle this epidemic of unnecessary treatment, which can lead to poor care for patients and escalating costs. National campaigns such as 'Too Much Medicine', 'Prudent Healthcare' and 'Choosing Wisely' have made important contributions to this debate. Their prime focus is on improving safety rather than decreasing costs, but they emphasize that waste can never be justified. I will return to these issues in the final chapter.

Costs are also driven up substantially by litigation, a hugely complex and emotive issue. In December 2015, a five-year-old British boy with cerebral palsy was awarded an £11.5 million settlement from the NHS. His brain had been deprived of oxygen in the womb when midwives at the hospital where he was born failed to notice that his mother's umbilical cord was prolapsed.[10] In 2016–17, parents made 232 legal claims against NHS trusts in England for severe birth injuries, up 23 per cent from the previous year. In September 2020, the former UK health secretary

Jeremy Hunt reported that the cost of litigation and compensation following poor care of mothers and babies was around £1 billion – almost twice the salary of all the labour doctors in England's hospitals combined.

In the National Health Service, litigation carries a quite extraordinary cost. In 2018, *The Times* reported that the NHS had paid £2.2 billion to settle negligence claims in the preceding year – a 30 per cent increase on the previous year – leading to renewed warnings that the cost of errors could end up crippling the service. Some £404 million of these costs were due to changes in the calculation of interest rates awarding bigger lump sums to people who required life-long care; even despite this, damages paid to claimants had increased by 13 per cent, to £1.2 billion.[11]

Identifying potential solutions for the causes of such massive figures is beyond the scope of this book, though there is clearly a vicious cycle at play. A cash-strapped service will inevitably struggle to deliver optimum quality, which results in problems and complaints, which lead to pay-outs, which result in less money being available for care. The solution must lie in addressing issues around staffing, education and quality. NHS Resolution, a body established to resolve concerns about healthcare fairly and efficiently, aims to challenge existing models of compensation, to keep cases out of the courts as far as possible, to minimize legal costs and to deliver resolution in its broadest sense, which is about more than just money.[12]

In the US, litigation costs can be astronomical. Even ten years ago, the cost of medical malpractice was about $55.6 billion a year – $45.6 billion of which was spent on defensive medicine practised by physicians desperate to avoid lawsuits.[13] The amount comprises 2.4 per cent of the nation's total healthcare expenditure.

The cost of drugs

But while healthcare expenses can be generated in all manner of ways, it tends to be drug costs that cause most controversy. As a 2018 report showed, prescription drugs are a very significant factor in healthcare costs. NHS spending on medicines in England grew from £13 billion in 2010–11 to £17.4 billion in 2016–17 – an average growth of around 5 per cent a year[14] – and it's not just the UK that is affected. Global expenditure on pharmaceuticals reached $1.135 trillion in 2017, up 56 per cent from 2007.[15]

The same report claimed that the rate of increase in pharmaceutical spending substantially outpaced the growth of the total NHS budget over the same period. Much of the recent growth in medicine spending had been in the hospital sector, where costs have grown at an average of 12 per cent a year since 2010–11.

The costs of individual drugs are only part of the story of escalating pharmaceutical costs, which also has demographic factors. Population growth and increases in the numbers of older people inevitably increase the volume of medicines required; older people are more likely to suffer from long-term health conditions such as cardiovascular problems, arthritis or diabetes,[16] which typically require lifelong treatment – prescriptions that are repeated month after month, year after year.

In addition, factors such as changing patient expectations, disease prevalence, pricing strategies and clinician behaviour can impact on cost. While some drugs are only prescribed in short courses – antibiotics being a prime example – a large number of drugs are used long term. Replacement therapies for hormonal conditions like an underactive thyroid gland or diabetes are prime examples.

In addition, overprescribing is a major issue. A report by the UK's chief pharmaceutical officer in 2021 estimated that 10 per cent of drugs were over-prescribed – that is, not needed or wanted by the patient, potentially more harmful than beneficial, or having more appropriate alternatives.[17]

This doesn't solely impact cost and waste. A fifth of hospital admissions in those aged over sixty-five are due to adverse effects of prescribed drugs, and 25 per cent of the NHS's carbon footprint comes from medicines.[18] As a family doctor, I lost count of the vast amounts of drugs that were returned to the surgery unopened, unused and apparently unwanted after a patient had died. There are complex reasons why patients continue to collect prescriptions and not take them, but the issue is one that has a profound impact.

Remarkably little research has been undertaken into when and how it is safe to discontinue taking drugs, meaning that many drugs end up being taken for decades. How can you decide when to stop taking a drug for a condition that is symptomless – raised cholesterol or high blood pressure, for example? Research into drug usage is largely paid for by the pharmaceutical companies, and it may not be rocket science to understand why they are more likely to fund research that promotes the need for patients to start taking their products rather than to stop taking them.

About five years ago, I began taking a particular medication with an expectation that I will take it twice a day for the rest of my life – assuming that science doesn't come up with a better alternative in the meantime. If I live to the average life expectancy of someone like me, living in my part of England, I will take approximately 12,000 of these tablets, and each one of them costs real money.

Let's multiply this up. A report by Dr Duncan Petty of the University of Bradford revealed that 43 per cent of the UK population are reliant on repeat prescriptions; over 800 million items of repeat medicines cost the NHS almost £8 billion a year – its biggest cost after staff and almost half its total spend on medicine. The report predicted that by 2039, 231 million more repeat prescriptions will be dispensed each year,[19] thanks in part to an increasingly elderly population. In 2017, it was estimated that by 2025, nearly one million more people will be living with long-term health conditions.

Pharmaceuticals
Long-term medication costs a huge amount of money, but short-term medication can also be breathtakingly expensive. The remainder of this chapter will focus on the cost of prescription pharmaceutical drugs – after all, it is these figures that so often hit the headlines, often alongside the question, 'Can we afford this new treatment?' The complex reality is that the money required for one person's potentially dangerous condition could benefit thousands of other people with less expensive conditions. How should we begin to tackle such an ethical dilemma?

I do not intend this chapter to be a rant about drug companies. Indeed, I believe – and have often said publicly – that society needs a strong and effective pharmaceutical industry. Many years ago, my brother John died from acute leukaemia at the tragically young age of thirty-eight. These days he would almost certainly have survived, thanks to drug treatments developed by the pharmaceutical industry. My father also died of heart disease when he was younger than I am now – I am certain that he would have lived far longer if current treatments had been available.

I also have no doubt that the pharmaceutical industry can be a force for good. Just look at the extraordinary impact that research and therapeutics have had on the treatment of HIV/AIDS – a condition that just a few years ago was seen as an inevitable death sentence is now eminently controllable, at least for those with access to drugs. I have met many fine and impressive people who work in the pharmaceutical industry. Their motivations are noble, and they want to make a difference. During the Covid-19 pandemic, the scientists who worked so hard to develop vaccines have been applauded publicly for their altruistic, life-saving achievements.

But in more typical times, the public perception of the pharmaceutical industry can be rather different. In any logical world, the professionals who develop new medications would be seen as core members of the healthcare team, along with doctors, nurses, pharmacists and the panoply of other staff who add value and care. However, those people who work in the pharmaceutical industry, far from being treated like the rest of the team, are instead denigrated and sneeringly described as 'Big Pharma'.

On typing the phrase 'Big Pharma' into an internet search engine, the first major article I reached carried the headline, 'Why Americans Hate Big Pharma More than Ever'.[20] The article revealed that a Gallup poll had 'found that the pharmaceutical sector is the most loathed industry in the country. It scored a net favorability rating of -31 points (27 per cent positive, 58 per cent negative), which is its lowest rating since the poll's inception in 2001.'

For an industry that is devoted to improving the health of humankind, this is a pretty extraordinary statistic, and to be regarded even less favourably than politicians is a remarkable achievement. However, the industry can be its own worst enemy, and I know that many people who work in it cringe at some of its behaviours.

A simple example relates to executive pay. According to reporting from Bloomberg, 'as drug giant Pfizer Inc. hiked the price of dozens of drugs in 2017, it also jacked up the compensation of CEO Ian Read by 61 per cent, putting his total compensation at $27.9

million ... Pfizer's board reportedly approved the compensation boost because they saw it as a "compelling incentive" to keep Read from retiring.'[21] Does that sound like a way to improve the image of such an important industry?

While most of us will look at such behaviour and ask what on earth they think they are doing, Pfizer's corporate aspirations, listed on their website, are entirely noble, including a commitment to global health, protecting people and the environment, and transparency. Is it just me who finds all this puzzling?

The cost of drugs is certainly one reason for the scepticism that many people feel towards the pharmaceutical industry. In August 2021, a report in *The Times* began, 'The pharmaceutical giant Pfizer and a British company have been accused of exploiting a loophole to charge the NHS "unfairly high" prices for an epilepsy drug that rose overnight from £2.83 to £67.50 per pack. The competition watchdog said that price rises of up to 2,600 per cent for phenytoin sodium capsules cost the NHS an extra £50 million a year.'[22]

In 2021, the UK's competition watchdog imposed fines of more than £100 million on the pharmaceutical company Advanz and its former private equity owners after it was found guilty of inflating the price of thyroid tablets by up to 6,000 per cent. According to a report in the *Guardian*, the price paid by the NHS for liothyronine tablets rose from £4.46 to £258.19 between 2007 and 2017, while production costs remained broadly stable.[23]

Or how about a September 2018 report from *The Sunday Times* with the headline 'Salary Size Matters, Says AstraZeneca Boss on £9.4m'? The article stated that Pascal Soriot, chief executive of the pharmaceuticals giant AstraZeneca, was annoyed that he was paid less than his peers. 'The truth is that I'm the lowest-paid CEO in the whole industry,' he said. 'It is annoying to some extent. But at the end of the day, that is what it is.' Perhaps the industry should consider whether there is any correlation between these astronomical salaries and the associated shareholder profits and the low esteem in which so many people hold it.

And nor are these isolated examples. The EpiPen is an auto-injector device containing adrenaline, which is used in severe allergic reactions to reverse low blood pressure, wheezing, skin itching, hives and other symptoms. Each year, about 3.6 million Americans are prescribed this drug. It is a wonderful development, and it saves lives.

In 2007, the pharmaceutical company Mylan acquired the right to market the EpiPen as part of its acquisition of Merck, and two years later the price began to steadily increase. In 2009, the wholesale price for a two-pack of auto-injectors was $103.50. By July 2013, the price was $264.50, and it rose a further 75 per cent by May 2015, to $461. By May 2016, the price was up to $608.61. Over a seven-year period, the price of EpiPens had risen by about 500 per cent.[24] It was hardly surprising that this led to a backlash from consumers and clinicians. I'll leave you to decide what might have motivated such behaviour – I know what I think.

It also seems that the pharmaceutical industry can be its own worst enemy. While many companies behave entirely ethically, those that exploit vulnerable patients are anything but. Price should be linked to value, not simply be set as high as the market can get away with. Faced with increasing drug costs, we need to know how they are justified, particularly at a time when perceptions of excessive profits and sky-high executive incomes are commonplace. And underlying many of these concerns is one key question.

How are drug prices calculated?

This should be a simple question to answer, but after several years of trying to unravel this issue – and I did warn you earlier that I am no health economist – the process remains a massive conundrum. No one has ever been prepared to give me a logical methodology for how any given drug is priced, in the way that it is possible to break down the price of other consumables.

For instance, a cup of coffee in a high-street coffee shop will inevitably have a massive profit margin when you consider how cheap it is to make at home, but it is nevertheless possible to examine the costs that contribute to the price you pay. The Speciality Coffee Association of America provided the following approximate breakdown of the cost of a double cappuccino:

Ingredients: 5 per cent
Dairy: 10 per cent
Cup/lid/sleeve: 2 per cent
Labour: 36 per cent
Rent: 10 per cent
Marketing: 5 per cent
General and administrative: 20 per cent
Operating profit: 11 per cent

When you try to conduct a similar analysis with even the most basic drugs, you hit a brick wall. The typical response from the pharmaceutical industry is that high costs are justified because of the high failure rate involved in developing new drugs and the massive cost of research. I understand that research is expensive and that years of development can come to nothing. As Sir Andrew Dillon, former chief executive of NICE, wrote in a letter to *The Times*, 'If it really does cost £1.2 billion to develop a new drug, the question the pharmaceutical industry must be able to answer is this: are you absolutely confident that it needs to?'[25]

Of course, I understand that such research has to be paid for and that there would be no new drugs without it, but I still don't understand how some levels of profit and remuneration can be morally justified. Even if we ignore the emotive issue of executive pay, our biggest challenge lies in working out what should be included in development costs. Raw ingredients and manufacturing costs tend to be relatively cheap, but research and development costs rapidly mount up. In addition, the R&D costs of the drugs that undergo the early stages of development but never get to market must also be factored in. Research companies need to cover the costs of these failed drugs and set them against the profits of the drugs that do work – this, they claim, is the only way in which they can afford to develop future medicines.

The Tufts Center for the Study of Drug Development has estimated that the current cost of developing a prescription drug is an astonishing $2.558 billion.[26] They based this figure on information obtained from ten pharma companies on 106 drugs, selected at random. The calculations are complex, but in essence, the costs of compounds abandoned during testing were linked to the costs of those that obtained marketing approval. The estimated average out-of-pocket cost for an approved new compound was $1,395 million, but the Tufts data showed that less than 12 per cent of drugs that enter the clinical pipeline are ever approved for marketing. It should also be noted that Tufts University declares that 25 per cent of its operating expenses come from the drugs industry and related companies,[27] and that an alternative analysis of ten new cancer drugs published in *JAMA Internal Medicine* put the median cost of such new drugs much lower, at $648 million – still a significant spend, but less than half the Tufts figure.[28]

Industry representatives have made it clear that without such investment and if the costs of failed products were not covered, the pipeline of life-saving drugs may well dry up. However, a significant number of products are invented in university laboratories where much of the funding comes from the public purse, with pharma companies buying the most promising products and then conducting larger-scale research and testing. A recent study in the US found that the National Institutes of Health contributed an average of $839 million in research for each of the 210 first-in-class drugs approved between 2010 and 2016.[29]

A report by Global Justice Now[30] showed that the UK government spent £2.3 billion on health R&D in 2015 alone. Globally, the report estimated that two-thirds of drug R&D costs are publicly funded, with around a third of all new medicines originating in public research institutions. On top of this, many medicines developed by pharmaceutical companies often benefit from work that has been paid for by the taxpayer.

However, the report also showed that even when the UK government funds a substantial proportion of the R&D for an innovative medicine, there is no guarantee either of an equitable public return on this public investment or that patients will be able to access the medicine at an affordable price. As a 2018 report in the *British Medical Journal* stated:

> Government funding for health innovation is subsidising drug industry profits while providing little public health benefit ... Most new drugs are not meeting public needs

while economic and regulatory incentives have created a 'highly inefficient pharmaceutical sector' which spends more on marketing than research and development, and focuses the research it does do on profits ... This leads to prohibitively high prices, but also to the side-lining of treatments aimed at prevention or cure in favour of drugs with long-term, high-volume sales potential.[31]

In a significant number of cases, the UK taxpayer is effectively paying for medicines twice: first through investment in R&D, and then by paying high prices for the medicine itself. Effectively, the report concluded, the commercialization of these discoveries has used public funds to generate huge private profits. A global system of intellectual property rights provides companies with time-limited monopolies, allowing them to charge high prices for products with relatively low production costs. If this is all true, the claims of pharmaceutical companies that these high prices are justified falls apart. If the public purse is funding a large proportion of the R&D, the justification for monopoly pricing is hard to sustain.

To add a further complexity, there is the law of diminishing returns. As each new drug is developed, it is compared with the current standard of care, which raises the bar for the next drug and makes it more expensive. In other words, the more we improve the standard of care, the more costly it will become to improve further. As a result, the pharmaceutical industry is spending more and more to achieve slighter benefits – hardly a sustainable business model.

As Billy Kenber writes in his powerful book *Sick Money*, 'you don't need to discover drugs to get rich from them anymore ... for many executives, pharmaceuticals have become little more than financial assets, to be flipped, dealt, exploited and manipulated in a myriad of creative and profitable ways'.[32]

Promotion and advertising

While pharmaceutical companies claim that their high costs are justified by the expense of research and development, many of them appear to spend just as much on sales and marketing as they do on R&D. A 2019 study in the *Journal of the American Medical Association* showed that spending on medical marketing increased from $17.7 billion to $29.9 billion between 1997 and 2016, with direct-to-consumer advertising for drugs and health services growing most rapidly, and marketing to health professionals accounting for most promotional spending.[33] The paper concluded:

> Increased medical marketing reflects a convergence of scientific, economic, legal and social forces. As more drugs and devices and medical advances convert once-fatal diseases into chronic illnesses and with renewed interest in prevention for some diseases, the marketing of tests, treatments and services has expanded. An ageing, more insured population, with Medicare Part D, the Affordable Care Act and a receptivity to lifestyle interventions, has expanded the customer reservoir. More clinicians, healthcare centers, for-profit sector growth and market consolidation have increased competition, stimulating marketing growth.

Whether the marketing of medication is a good thing is another matter entirely, but it has certainly been a powerful driver of escalating cost, not to mention profit. As Jerry Avorn, a professor of medicine at Harvard Medical School, wrote in the *New York Times*, 'this advertising promotes only the most expensive products, it drives prescription costs up and also encourages the "medicalization" of American life – the sense that pills are needed for most everyday problems'.[34] Is it any wonder that healthcare costs are spiralling out of control?

Patents

Prices are also maintained by patent laws, which prevent competing manufacturers making copycat drugs and pushing the price down. Drug patents apply for twenty years and must be registered in each country where the product is used. Once the patent runs out, however, costs can drop dramatically. In the UK, the NHS saved £110 million by implementing a policy to use the best-value adalimumab (a drug used to treat various types of arthritis) after the brand-name medication Humira lost European patent protection. Although there is little doubt that savings can be made from these sorts of policies, it takes time for the cheaper versions of drugs to come on the market – and in the patent-covered phase, costs remain eye-wateringly high.

Another major factor that impacts on drug pricing is the relatively small potential market for many of the newer drugs. Over the last twenty years or so, research and development has increasingly moved away from developing simple drugs that target widespread chronic diseases, the development costs of which could be spread over many millions of patients. Instead, the drugs that are developed now are more often large, complex molecules that, while dramatically effective, often target much smaller patient populations.

Drugs used for conditions that only small numbers of patients suffer from are sometimes described as 'orphan drugs'. They would not be profitable to produce without government assistance, being designed to treat conditions that are referred to as 'orphan diseases'. Between 1990 and 1995, the US Food and Drug Administration approved between fifty-five and eighty-nine drug company requests for orphan drug disease status each year. Over the last few years, the number of such requests has escalated, with the FDA granting this status to 260 molecules in 2013 and 293 in 2014.

International implications

Another complex issue relates to the cost of drugs on the international market. What are the ethics of charging a price that is unaffordable for any low- and middle-income country? Conversely, if drugs are sold much more cheaply in these countries, what would stop them being sold to richer countries at a profit, but a price that makes the drugs more affordable for the richer countries, while depriving the poorer countries of therapeutic benefits?

In 2016, the UN produced a report looking at these issues.[35] As the press release to accompany it said, 'Whether it's the rising price of the EpiPen or new outbreaks of diseases like Ebola, Zika and yellow fever, the rising costs of health technologies and the lack of new tools to tackle health problems, like antimicrobial resistance, is a problem in rich and poor countries alike.'

As the report explained, international treaties and national constitutions have for decades enshrined the fundamental right to health, as well as the right to share the benefits of scientific advancements. Yet while the world is witnessing the immense potential of science and technology, many countries and communities are suffering from major gaps and failures in the treatment of disease. Tension is fuelled by a misalignment between the right to health on the one hand and intellectual property and trade on the other. This is perhaps inevitable when profit is the driving force behind development.

The UN report formulated a set of concrete recommendations to improve people's access to vital therapies that are currently unaffordable for patients and governments. Unsurprisingly, it confirmed that the cost of health technologies is putting a strain on rich and poor countries alike.

Malebona Precious Matsoso, director general of the South African National Department of Health and one of the report's authors, gave a statement in which she called for change:

> With no market incentives, there is an innovation gap in diseases that predominantly affect neglected populations, rare diseases and a crisis particularly with antimicrobial resistance, which poses a threat to humanity. Our report calls on governments to negotiate global agreements on the coordination, financing and development of health technologies to complement existing innovation models, including a binding R&D convention that delinks the costs of R&D from end prices.

Delinking the costs of research and development from the end price of treatments would only be possible if a deal could be worked out that rewarded companies for developing a drug without them needing to depend on sales. Indeed, recent work around the need for new antibiotics has taken this approach; if the world is to avoid the perils of antimicrobial resistance, the use of any new antibiotic must be highly restricted. This is not the typical model of sales that the pharmaceutical industry depends on, but one that the world absolutely needs.

Discounts

Drug pricing is further complicated by the substantial discounts that may be given to institutional purchasers of medicines, following negotiation. Such confidential discounts are widely used in high-income countries and can vary considerably across therapeutic areas and between countries.[36] However, the major problem with such discounts is that each nation or payer negotiates without knowing the price paid by others, and the wealthiest countries are likely to be the toughest negotiators. Perversely, those with a greater need may end up paying more. Keeping final prices secret effectively prevents everyone from demanding the lowest available price. There is already evidence that some medications are more expensive in low- and middle-income countries than in wealthy countries.[37] Does that sound like a just solution?

Profits

While we should be grateful for many of the products developed by the pharmaceutical industry, it remains an extraordinarily profitable business. According to Proclinical, the most profitable global pharmaceutical companies in 2019 were:

1. Pfizer – $53.7 billion
2. Roche – $45.6 billion
3. Johnson & Johnson – $40.7 billion
4. Sanofi – $39.3 billion
5. Merck – $37.7 billion
6. Novartis – $34.9 billion
7. AbbVie – $32.8 billion
8. Amgen – $23.7 billion

9. GlaxoSmithKline – $23 billion
10. Bristol Myers Squibb – $22.6 billion[38]

It is little wonder that these companies are attractive to investors. A while ago, I met a major investor at a meeting about drug pricing. He was clear that investors were generally 'ethically neutral' – return was what they valued most.

Covid-19

The extraordinary, rapid and life-saving development of the Covid-19 vaccines is one of the great success stories of our age. However, as a report in *The Times* pointed out, while governments committed billions of pounds of investment, and publicly funded scientists had been working on vaccine developments for years, 'the trillion-dollar commercial industry largely viewed responding to outbreaks and developing vaccines for diseases afflicting poor countries as incompatible with their profit-driven ethos'.[39]

According to one example in this report, the value of Moderna – a Boston biotech firm – soared from $6.5 billion to more than $180 billion, but the development of its vaccine was fully funded by the US government. Meanwhile AstraZeneca was ultimately persuaded by scientists at the Jenner Institute in Oxford that their vaccine should be sold on a not-for-profit basis. The company agreed to make several billion doses available at cost while the pandemic lasted and to supply lower-income countries at that price indefinitely. By November 2020, this laudable and humane approach had resulted in a 3.8 per cent fall in share price, a decline of $4 billion in the company's value.[40]

As a report in *Forbes* magazine succinctly concluded, 'The pandemic crisis offered a challenge that government might have used to restructure the shareholder model of for-profit medicine, a model that dates to the 1980s and corporate America's turn toward putting shareholders above the public good. Instead, taxpayer money flowed to a small group of capitalists with almost no strings attached and little transparency.'[41]

Of course we should be immensely grateful for the vaccines. Of course we should praise to the skies the scientists who worked on these life-saving products. They were magnificent. But are the profit levels of the companies in any way justified? According to *Forbes*, seven Pfizer executives made $14 million in stock sales in 2020, while Moderna executives made $287 million in stock sales in the same year. I deliberately used the word 'made' rather than 'earned'. This is no way for the industry to earn the respect that it so craves.

Cancer

The drugs that are used to treat cancer have had a profound impact on the lives of many of us who would previously have succumbed, but they are also quite extraordinarily expensive. The analysis group Evaluate Pharma estimated that sales of oncology medicines were $123.8 billion in 2018 (out of a total prescription medicine market of $864 billion), while a report released in 2016 put worldwide spending on cancer drugs at $107 billion. A disproportionate amount of this money – some 45 per cent – is spent in the United States.

These drugs are certainly profitable. In a study of ninety-nine cancer drugs approved by the US Food and Drugs Administration between 1989 and 2017, the median income return by the end of 2017 was $14.50 for every dollar spent on research and development.[42] As the paper concluded, 'Cancer drugs, through high prices, have generated returns for the originator companies far in excess of possible R&D costs. Lowering prices of cancer drugs and facilitating greater competition are essential for improving patient access, health system's financial sustainability and future innovation.'

As a report in the *Journal of Oncology* stated, 'In the context of cancer therapy, the prices of new anti-cancer agents seem to be decided by pharmaceutical companies according to what the market will bear. There is little correlation between the actual efficacy of a new drug and its price, as measured by cost-efficacy ratios, prolongation of patient life in years or quality-adjusted life-years.'[43]

The challenge doesn't end there. A 2017 paper in the *British Medical Journal* threw up a stark challenge. An evaluation of oncology approvals by the European Medicines Agency between 2009 and 2013 showed that most drugs entered the market without there being any evidence of them benefiting either survival or quality of life. Indeed, at a minimum of 3.3 years after they had gone on sale, there was no conclusive evidence that these drugs either extended or improved life for most cancer patients – and where there were survival gains over existing treatment options or a placebo, they were often marginal.[44] As one responder wrote, 'The article gives voice to many medical oncologists and haematologists around the world who are alarmed by the escalating cost system without significant demonstration of efficacy and cost-effectiveness.'

Just to complicate matters further, new generations of cancer drugs are simultaneously becoming much more effective and even more expensive. Chimeric antigen receptor T-cell therapy involves taking extracts of the patient's own white blood cells, which are re-engineered to recognize and attack cancer cells before being infused back into the patient. These treatments are extraordinarily expensive, not least because they are specific to each individual.

Such is the efficacy of some cancer drugs now that some patients for whom treatment would previously have been impossible can be successfully treated. As an example, a drug called tisagenlecleucel was assessed in the UK as being suitable for up to 200 patients with relapsed or refractory diffuse large B-cell lymphoma. This is a form of cancer of the lymphatic system, the series of lymph glands and the fine tubes that join them throughout the body. Its list price is £282,000 and it is given as a single intravenous infusion. Drugs like this are fantastic and life-changing; as a result of them, conditions that were previously untreatable will potentially be vanquished. So how do we afford them?

A paper in *Nature Reviews Clinical Oncology* stated that the lifetime cost of treatment for a single patient with chronic lymphocytic leukaemia was predicted to rise by 310 per cent between 2011 and 2025, from $147,000 to $604,000. When coupled with a growth in the prevalence of this condition, the increase would push US spending from an estimated $0.74 billion to $5.13 billion for this type of cancer alone.[45,46]

With prices at this level, it is no wonder that no health system can afford to make every new anti-cancer drug available to every patient who might need it. When the patient must cover some or all of the cost, price rises can cause significant harm, with a large number of patients delaying or skipping treatment. People who don't take their drugs as advised are far more likely to require hospitalization at a later point, which adds to the overall cost of care.

As the costs of anti-cancer drugs continue to increase, it will only be a matter of time before they become unsustainable. If there was a straightforward correlation between price and value – as there is around almost everything else – the discussion would be much easier to understand. We can't go on like this.

CHAPTER 5

Valuing a Life

Anyone who is fortunate enough to live in a country with comprehensive state-funded healthcare is unlikely to have any idea what their medicines really cost. Although some drugs can be very cheap – aspirin, for example, has been around since 1899 and costs just a few pence – other drugs are extraordinarily expensive, as we have already seen. In the UK, it is often only when people take their pet to the vet and have to pay for its medication, or if they fall ill while on a foreign holiday and receive a bill for emergency treatment, that the true cost of pharmaceuticals really hits them – and it usually comes as something of a shock.

Ignorance may be bliss, but we need to remember that half of the UK population take at least one prescription drug every day,[1] and the figure is similar in the US.[2] A quarter of people in the UK are on at least three drugs, with millions, particularly the elderly, on at least five types of medication. These costs really add up. For instance, in one recent year the net ingredient cost of atorvastatin, the most prescribed statin in the UK, was £52,621,269, the cost of levothyroxine sodium (a treatment for an underactive thyroid gland) was £86,942,415 and the cost of omeprazole (a treatment that reduces stomach acid) was £52,767,333. These are quite remarkable numbers.[3] The trouble is that, as we have seen elsewhere, they are so massive that they have little real meaning.

But it's not just these cumulative figures that cause the huge expense, for the cost of individual doses can also be breathtakingly high. As I mentioned in Chapter 1, in May 2019 the FDA in the United States approved Zolgensma, then the most expensive treatment in history. It was a treatment for spinal muscular atrophy, a rare disorder caused by a defective gene that weakens a child's muscles so dramatically that they become unable to move and eventually unable to swallow or breathe. In the US, it occurs in about 400 babies each year.

This therapy was priced at $2.125 million per patient by Novartis, who argued that spread across a lifetime, this price was cost-effective. Novartis did not develop Zolgensma themselves but had bought AveXis, the company that did. The *Wall Street Journal* described the acquisition as a 'bet', with the high price necessary for that gamble to be successful.[4]

Other 2019 drug prices in the US (based on the price for one month's treatment) include:

Actimmune: $52,321.80
Daraprim: $45,000
Cinryze: $44,140.64
Chenodal: $42,570

The price of drugs is putting increasing pressure on every health system in the world. In 2017, NHS England reported that its drugs bill had grown annually by over 7 per cent, a considerably faster rate of growth than the change in the overall NHS budget. Faced with figures like these, what can possibly be done about cost, and in particular about expensive new products, many of which are exciting new compounds with real potential? How can healthcare systems and individuals cope?

Price and value

Let us consider for a moment how price affects other purchases. I would love to own a Mercedes-Benz, and particularly the top-of-the-range S-Class Coupé. I've never driven one, but I can tell from the brochure that it would suit me just fine. The problem? It costs a mere £187,560. There is no way that I would ever choose a car like that, so the solution is simple. I will stick to my excellent – and economically priced – Skoda. If you can't afford something, you can't have it.

Logically, these rules would apply to healthcare, too. You get whatever you, or whoever is paying, can afford. But what if you get a rare, potentially fatal but treatable disease, but the medication is unaffordable? If you live in a society where your only option is to pay directly for your own care, the answer is relatively straightforward, if a little cruel. You either beg, borrow, steal or earn the money, or you succumb to the disease. It's a choice between 'Your money or your life,' a question that Dick Turpin and his fellow highwaymen are reputed to have asked.

But if society is paying for your care through taxation, how does it go about making these decisions? How does it decide that providing you with the Mercedes S-Class of care is a justified expense? Recognizing that every pound or dollar can only be spent once, how does society decide that spending all that money on you is worthwhile? After all, if it is, it can no longer be spent on someone else. Who should get the care? When should we say no? Should a small number of people get a new Mercedes, while others have to put up with a second-hand banger? Is it better for a few people to have a wonderful car, or for everyone to have an average one?

If you live in a country where your care is covered by an insurance policy, the companies that pay for your care will be interested in this debate. After all, no one has infinite funds – perhaps other than the mega-rich tech tycoons of Silicon Valley and the occasional oligarch. In the real world, there are limits to how much can be afforded. I recall visiting one South American country where a senior executive of a health insurance company said, 'If the government won't bite the bullet and take action on drug costs, we'll have to do it. We simply can't go on like this. We can't afford to, and if we put our premiums up to cover these prices, our customers won't be able to afford them.' This debate is important for everyone, however your healthcare is funded.

I recently discussed these issues with a colleague from a country that provides universal health coverage, despite not being one of the most affluent of nations. This country has recently struggled with an issue relating to a class of highly expensive medicines. A form of these medicines that is just as effective but dramatically cheaper is now available, but the makers of the expensive drugs are encouraging doctors and patients to demand their more costly therapies, with the country's supreme court ruling that patients have an absolute right to them. The law, on this occasion, is ignoring the human rights of the citizens who either will not receive care or whose treatment will be delayed because much-needed funds have been wasted on an unnecessarily expensive therapy.

It is a hugely complex and emotive topic. Unfortunately, discussion of cost control in the US is often met with talk of 'death panels', mythical organizations of faceless bureaucrats who 'choose who lives and who dies'. If such organizations existed we would have grounds for concern, but the reality is simple: unless we accept every single drug or product produced by every single pharmaceutical company for use at any price, someone has to be responsible for making decisions about what is reasonable and what isn't. After all, we make similar decisions about everything else we buy. When you were considering whether to buy this book, you probably weighed up how much it cost and how interesting it looked before making your choice. Had the publisher priced it at £200, you would have snorted and put it straight back on the shelf – and rightly so. Prices matter and benefits have to be justified – even in healthcare. But the debate might feel rather different if your life ever depends on a hyper-expensive drug.

If this thought is making you feel uncomfortable, consider an entirely fictional new drug called Pharmalidomide, developed to treat a rare form of cancer. The manufacturers claim that it helps extend the life of those suffering from this life-threatening condition, but to take it for a single year would cost £250,000. You may be thinking that a quarter of a million pounds is nothing compared to dying – if you were faced with the cost, you would do anything to find the money. Indeed, if you live somewhere with universal health coverage, you would expect the state to pay for the cost of your care. But what if the average additional survival time was only four months, and there was a high chance that someone taking this drug would spend most of this extra time feeling severely nauseated and profoundly weak? Would it still be worth it? And what if the drug's side effects were continual diarrhoea and insomnia?

If you live in a country with an insurance-funded healthcare system, what would your attitude be to the cost of Pharmalidomide? If your insurance scheme pays the full cost of the drug for anyone who needs it, the chances are that your premiums would increase. Do you still think it is good value? You might think it justified to spend that money on you or your family, but would you feel the same if it was for someone you'd never met, or the homeless man you saw on the street this morning? Would that make any difference?

You might think all this talk of cost is obscene, but let me press you further. Imagine the drug now costs £500,000. Is it still worth it? And what if it cost vastly more – perhaps £25,000,000 per year. Would it still be worth it? Indeed, do you think there is any limit on how much should be paid for a drug that – for instance – adds just six months to someone's life?

If there is any point at which you find yourself saying, 'No, an extra six months isn't worth that much,' then you are indicating that you think the cost of treatment is a factor that should be taken into consideration. The debate then becomes about the price and not the principle. Some people might see this as 'rationing', but I prefer to describe it as 'being rational' – a better option than being irrational.

Tough decisions

Tough decisions need to be made. During the worst early days of the coronavirus crisis, it became clear in many European countries that demand for ventilators was outstripping supply. In this situation, choices had to be made. Inevitably, there was anxiety, particularly across social media, that one group or another was being written off – whether because of age, infirmity, learning disability or another factor. I recently spent a depressing hour reading the comments posted on Twitter while #DNACPR (which stands for 'do not attempt cardiopulmonary resuscitation') was trending. I could understand why people might be fearful that doctors had written them off without them having any say in the matter.

In the vast majority of situations, such directives regarding cardiopulmonary resuscitation, far from being imposed, should be developed in partnership with patients. But as the chair of the

British Medical Association's medical ethics committee wrote in the *Guardian* during the crisis:

> Despite heroic efforts to increase supply – and reduce demand – there may come a point when this tsunami will simply overwhelm intensive-care beds, ventilators and life-support machines. Although we hope this will not happen, it is important we begin to think now about how we would respond should that situation arise. As in Spain and Italy, heart-wrenching decisions may need to be made, agonising choices about who gets access to life-saving interventions. Should there be a disjunction between need and resource, these decisions will become unavoidable. The question is how do we ensure decisions made are ethical?[5]

The committee issued a set of guidelines to help clinicians facing these remarkably challenging decisions that recognized the absolute importance of fairness.[6] However, if everyone matters equally but it is not possible to treat all those who require care, how can resources be allocated fairly?

In times of plenty, we allocate resources according to medical need. In most healthcare systems, it has long been clear that the more serious your illness, the greater the urgency with which you are treated. However, when we were faced with a global pandemic, this approach was overturned. The question was no longer how we could best meet individual need, but how we could maximize the benefits from severely stretched resources. To the criterion of medical need, we must also add the likelihood that the patient will benefit. If a number of patients have the same level of need, is it preferable to treat those who have a high likelihood of benefiting than those who have a low chance of benefiting? The principle that everyone matters is in tension with the requirement to maximize overall benefit, but as the BMA report observed, this was at the heart of the debate.

Coronavirus simply highlighted the challenge that healthcare systems around the world have long faced. How do you make difficult decisions that attempt to balance cost and benefit? Let us return to our exorbitant invented drug Pharmalidomide, and the question I posed about whether you would take it if it offered some benefits but significant side effects. If you are the patient who might benefit and money is no object, the decision is yours alone. In my experience, the way in which people approach such decisions varies a great deal. For some, the thought of a few extra months, however dreadful the quality of life, is seen as worth it, particularly if they have a future event that they would like to attend – a family wedding, perhaps, or the birth of a grandchild.

Other people, even if they can easily afford the treatment, will choose to place a greater value on the quality of life than on the length of time they live for. I've been particularly intrigued by the case of Wilko Johnson, the former guitarist with the British rock band Dr Feelgood. In 2013, on being diagnosed with terminal pancreatic cancer, he chose not to undertake chemotherapy, instead vowing to 'rock on for as long as possible' and to 'party where he can'.[7] While the prognosis turned out to be dramatically better than he was initially told and he was able to make a full recovery, it was his reaction when he expected the worst that fascinated me. For him, a farewell tour in front of adoring fans was infinitely more appealing than a course of radiotherapy and chemotherapy. Until we are faced with such a challenge, none of us know how we would respond. Does length of life trump everything else, or is quality of life what matters most? As the famous quotation goes, 'Life is not measured by the number of breaths you take but by the moments that take your breath away.'

For those of us who depend on funding for our treatment from elsewhere – whether it is paid for by the state or covered by insurance – the debate is equally complex. If the cost of the drug comes from the public purse, we need to ensure that the benefits of the treatment are justified by the cost. Insurance companies do not have infinite purses either, and they are left facing some very tricky decisions.

In the US, healthcare costs are a significant cause of bankruptcy – though the actual figures are a matter of considerable debate.[8,9] However, whatever the true figure, there is no doubt that people can be left struggling by excessive costs – it is not an issue we can pretend does not exist.

Some people think the subject is too toxic to be discussed, but they should realize that considering this challenging matter is a million miles away from the concept of death panels. As Sarah Palin wrote on Facebook in August 2009:

> The Democrats promise that a government healthcare system will reduce the cost of healthcare, but as the economist Thomas Sowell has pointed out, government healthcare will not reduce the cost; it will simply refuse to pay the cost. And who will suffer the most when they ration care? The sick, the elderly and the disabled, of course. The America I know and love is not one in which my parents or my baby with Down syndrome will have to stand in front of Obama's 'death panel' so his bureaucrats can decide, based on a subjective judgement

of their 'level of productivity in society', whether they are worthy of healthcare. Such a system is downright evil.[10]

I absolutely agree that such a system would indeed be evil, if that was what an organization that examined value in healthcare actually did. Unfortunately, every time questions around cost and value are raised in the US in relation to healthcare, the term 'death panels' tends to resurface, at the expense of an important public debate.

As this book has already demonstrated, in a world where there is more demand for healthcare than there are resources to pay for it, decisions on value are inevitable. If we ask whether money should be spent on something of minimal value for patient A if it results in patient B not getting vital treatment, this isn't a death panel – it is the very opposite. If not paying exorbitant prices for cancer drugs that aren't especially effective means that more money is available to treat patients with mental health problems, this is a very real benefit.

No matter what it costs …

Any decisions that are taken in this area are inevitably hugely controversial. As a letter to the *Northern Echo* in the UK stated:

> Here we go again, I refer to the article 'Cancer drug will not be funded'. The National Institute for Health and Care Excellence (NICE) stated that 'it would like to recommend Dinutuximab Beta for inclusion in the Cancer Drugs Fund (CDF) but it was too expensive to do so'. It is evidently estimated that this same drug would cost the NHS thousands of pounds in treating people for neuroblastoma cancer (which could enable cancer patients to live a bit longer) … So, which is

important – money or human life? If a drug is available to help people with a painful and life-threatening disease (no matter the cost), then the drug (or drugs) should be available on the NHS.[11]

There is no one who won't understand that argument, but think again about the phrase 'no matter the cost' and try to take away the emotion. How do we apply that idea and treat everyone who wants care without an infinite budget? And incidentally, following the rejection of this cancer drug by NICE on cost grounds, the pharmaceutical company involved negotiated a lower price that allowed it to be used. If the price hadn't been considered, the company would have been allowed to charge the original asking price, and other people would have missed out on funding for treatment. Many people believe that analysing price and cost-effectiveness are unethical, but I believe the exact opposite, especially in a publicly funded system. Surely the unethical act is to ignore the value, price and cost-effectiveness of a drug?

So how might we decide what is good value and what isn't? The simplest way would be to look at survival time. You could ask how much a drug costs and by how long it extends the patient's life. A simple sum could give you a score in pounds or dollars per extra month or year of life.

But would this be fair? Imagine two drugs have exactly the same price and are used to treat the same condition. Drug A results in patients living for an extra five years, during which they feel normal, with no symptoms whatsoever. Drug B also results in patients living for an extra five years, but they spend much of it feeling dreadful – with nausea, headaches, exhaustion and a multiplicity of other symptoms. Both drugs give the same length of life, so are they equally valuable? If you were paying for them out of your own money, I would be very surprised if you thought they each represented the same value for money.

For this reason, many organizations that are charged with making decisions regarding the cost-effectiveness of treatments use a methodology that combines the length and the quality of life. It is known as the 'quality-adjusted life year', and while it isn't perfect, it is a way of calculating whether treatments add value. As my examples of drugs A and B show, the differences between treatments can be very significant, and we need to work out a way of demonstrating them.

Measuring the quantity of life is easy – after all, someone is either alive or dead. If we know the date when a diagnosis was made or a treatment was started and the date on which that patient died, we have a clear way of measuring survival in years, months or days.

When it comes to quality of life, measurement is much harder. There are numerous different approaches, but the most straightforward one tries to measure quality on a spectrum between zero (dead) and one (perfect health). This score is often measured in terms of someone's ability to go about their daily life, and their freedom from pain and mental disturbance. How are you feeling today on this scale? If your score is one, I'm envious; while I'm delighted to be alive, I have all manner of aches and pains that would prevent me from scoring a full house. This score (which for me would be 0.8, at least today) is the utility value.

While this might sound straightforward, the more one thinks about it, the more complex it becomes. After all, the definition of perfect health is extremely subjective. The World Health Organization defines it as a 'state of complete physical, mental and social wellbeing, and not merely the absence of disease or infirmity'.

Have you ever felt that good? And how would that affect your scoring?

The quality-adjusted life year, or QALY, was invented in the 1970s and is now used around the world. A QALY score is calculated by multiplying years of life by utility value. In other words, if someone lives in perfect health for a year, they will have a QALY score of one; if they live in perfect health for six months, they will have a QALY score of 0.5. By contrast, if someone lives for a full year but with a much less good quality of life (a 0.5 utility score), they will also have a QALY score of 0.5.

One year of perfect life is thus rated as being the same as two years of life that are 50 per cent perfect. Although it's not without its faults, it recognizes that surviving for longer is not the only thing that matters, and as such can be used to measure the quality and quantity of life that someone may gain from a new treatment.

Organizations in many countries use the QALY as a means of determining whether a new treatment brings the benefits that it may claim. One of the first organizations to carry out what are known as 'health technology assessments' was England's National Institute for Clinical Excellence – which is now called the National Institute for Health and Care Excellence, a recognition of its broadening scope in public health and social care.

When looking at a new treatment, NICE compares it with the current best treatment to determine if there is a benefit. The current standard of care is used as the baseline, before the QALYs gained from the new treatment are calculated.

As an example, if a person currently typically lives for three years with a condition, and the best current treatment results in a utility value of 0.7, then this individual will have 2.1 QALYs. A pharmaceutical company may then develop a new treatment – let's call it Bettolol – which, although it doesn't increase life expectancy, is claimed to have fewer side effects. In tests, it becomes clear that the utility value has increased to 0.9 – the patient will now have 2.7 QALYs. In comparing the new treatment with existing best treatment, its benefit will be counted as 0.6 QALYs (2.1 subtracted from 2.7).

Now let's imagine that another company develops another new medicine called Extralol that treats the same condition. Trials show that it prolongs the patient's life by two years at a utility level of 0.7, so this new medicine benefits the patient with 1.4 additional QALYs.

What is the point of all this, and how do the QALY scores help? Well, by calculating and costing, they can help to unravel the dilemma faced by healthcare providers. There is a constant stream of new and expensive drugs, and we somehow need to determine whether their cost is justified by the benefits they bring. Of course, the QALY is not on its own sufficient to tell you if a treatment provides good value for money compared with current treatments – it must be assessed in combination with the cost of the new medicine, which produces a ratio called the 'cost per QALY'.

Imagine a patient has a potentially terminal condition and is receiving a treatment called WonderDrug. If they continue with this drug, it is known that they will probably live for ten years with a quality of life that is about half as good as normal (0.5). If a similar patient is instead given HyperDrug, research shows that they are likely to live for twelve years with a quality of life that is 75 per cent normal (0.75).

To compare HyperDrug with WonderDrug, you can look at the QALYs that have been gained: WonderDrug scores five QALYs (ten years x 0.5), while HyperDrug scores nine QALYs (twelve years x

0.75). However, although HyperDrug results in four additional QALYs, it costs an additional £100,000.

The final calculation is to divide the difference in treatment cost by the number of QALYs a treatment gains, in order to work out the cost per QALY. In this example, HyperDrug would cost £25,000 per QALY. This is information that NICE can use to assess its value for money. If a drug cost £50,000 more than the alternative and only gave the patient six months more life in good health, it would cost £100,000 per QALY gained. Or if another new drug with the same price gave the patient two more years of life in good health, it would cost £25,000 per QALY gained.

However, there are significant benefits that might not necessarily be captured by the QALY score; for this reason, the final decisions of NICE are made by committees of humans, including patients and clinical experts, who have the capacity to use their judgement. If this was not helpful, an algorithm would be all that was required.

Although these issues are under constant review, NICE has in the past stated that it considers interventions that cost the NHS less than £20,000 per QALY gained to be cost-effective, while those that cost up to £30,000 per QALY gained might be considered cost-effective if certain conditions are satisfied. On occasion, particularly for drugs that are used to treat very rare conditions, the threshold can be much higher.

The cut-off point for such decisions is complex. If you set it too high, many patients will be denied therapy. But if you set it too low, while the healthcare system may save money, the pharmaceutical industry may be discouraged from developing new products. Karl Claxton, professor of health economics at the University of York, has argued that NICE's threshold should be dropped significantly; he claims that if we stopped spending money on drugs that cost more than £13,000 per quality-adjusted life year, this would improve health outcomes overall for the NHS.[12]

While I don't wish to get into the complexities of an academic discussion of health economics, I believe two things are clear. Firstly, it is possible to design a robust and logical methodology to tackle the extraordinarily complex ethical issues facing our healthcare systems around cost and value. And secondly, society needs to give more attention to where our overall priorities should lie.

NICE has also recognized that not everything can be covered by scientific evidence and clinical trials. It also takes into account the values of the society in which it operates, which vary from country to country. In addition, for the past few years NICE has been part of a research project – 'Extending the QALY' – investigating how quality-of-life measures can be extended into areas of social care and public health and evaluating new ways of assessing the quality of health and wellbeing.

The difficult decisions about cost-effectiveness are made not by NICE employees but by independent committees known as technology appraisal committees, whose members are drawn from the NHS, patient and carer organizations, academia and the pharmaceutical and medical devices industries. Although these committees seek the views of organizations that represent health professionals, patients, carers, manufacturers and the government, their advice is independent of any vested interests. In addition, NICE subscribes to the following widely accepted moral principles that generally underpin clinical and public health practice:[13]

Respect for autonomy. This recognizes the rights of individuals to make informed choices about healthcare, health promotion and health protection, and from it arises the concept of 'patient choice'.

This moral principle cannot be applied universally – for example, some people may be unable to make informed choices because of mental or physical incapacity, while some public health measures (such as a ban on smoking in enclosed spaces) must be imposed on whole populations.

Non-maleficence. This involves an obligation not to inflict harm – either physical or psychological. Of course, as any treatment can have adverse consequences, it may be necessary to balance the benefits and harms when considering a particular intervention.

Beneficence. This involves an obligation to benefit individuals, but no clinical or public health intervention is beneficial for everyone. In the context of the work of NICE, the balancing of benefits and harms is usually more relevant.

Distributive justice. The mismatch between demands and resources leads to the problem of allocating limited resources fairly. There are, broadly speaking, two approaches that can be taken in publicly funded healthcare systems. The first is the utilitarian approach, which involves allocating resources to maximize the health of the community. This allows an efficient distribution of resources, but it can also lead the interests of minorities to be overridden by the majority, and it may not help in eradicating health inequalities. Alternatively, the egalitarian approach involves distributing the healthcare resources to allow each individual to have a fair share. It allows an adequate level of healthcare, but raises questions as to what is 'fair' and cannot be fully applied when resources are limited.

You could endlessly debate which approach is the more ethical basis for the allocation of resources; instead, NICE seeks to apply the same principles that underpin the NHS, through an emphasis on 'procedural justice'. The processes by which decisions are reached are transparent, as are the reasons for them. NICE does almost everything in public, unless there are commercially sensitive reasons that necessitate confidentiality. Indeed, its board – which I was privileged to chair for six years – even holds its meetings in public and encourages participation from any member of the public who wants to attend. It seemed to me that transparency was the best way of generating trust in public institutions, which is generally in short supply.

For this reason, when I'm asked to advise governments around the world about how they might set up similar organizations, I always emphasize the importance of transparency – without it, patients, the public and journalists will be suspicious as to the reasons for particular decisions. Any conflicts of interest must be tackled openly – it is inappropriate, for example, for clinicians who receive funding from a pharmaceutical company to be involved in decisions regarding products from that company, and the same goes for members of patient organizations that are funded by the pharmaceutical company concerned.

People may disagree with the decisions made by NICE, but they should at least understand that logical and transparent processes have been followed. It is vital that organizations like NICE are fully accountable – the citizens who pay for the NHS should have the opportunity to be involved in the allocation of the service's resources. The operations of NICE are very much more complex than this brief summary implies, including a modified methodology known as the Cancer Drugs Fund, designed for drugs for use in cancer but about which there is significant remaining clinical uncertainty that needs further investigation through data collection in the NHS or clinical studies. In this situation, NICE approves funding for the drug, in order to avoid long delays, but stresses the need for more information on its effectiveness before it can be considered for routine use.

I hope that I've demonstrated some of the ways in which these extraordinarily difficult decisions can be taken. When newspapers report that NICE has chosen not to approve a drug, this is not a decision that has been taken lightly by the 'pointy-headed bean counters', as a national newspaper once asserted.

It is also clear that methodologies like QALY scores are quite crude; it is more than likely that we will eventually have more sophisticated tools with which to tackle these complex issues. Though not a perfect system by any means, QALYs are currently the best available way of bringing together length of survival, quality and cost in one simple number. These are important issues that we cannot ignore; in societies in which policymakers and individuals have to make decisions around prioritization, they allow the cost-efficiency of different forms of healthcare intervention to be compared.

As the World Health Organization has made clear, every healthcare system faces problems of justice and efficiency related to the allocation of a limited pool of resources to a population.[14] Different countries tackle the issue of cost-effectiveness in a variety of ways. Like NICE, organizations such as IQWIG in Germany, HITAP in Thailand, HAS in France and NECA in South Korea all try to make fair choices. Australia has the Pharmaceutical Benefits Advisory Committee, an independent expert body appointed by the Australian government and including doctors, health professionals, health economists and consumer representatives among its members. Its primary role is to recommend new medicines that should be listed on Australia's Pharmaceutical Benefits Scheme. No new medicine can be listed without a positive recommendation from the committee.

New Zealand has a similar body, the Pharmaceutical Management Agency, which describes its role with beautiful simplicity: 'We work hard to give New Zealanders access to medicines and medical equipment they need to live healthy lives. Medicines and medical equipment can cost a lot of money. We have a fixed budget to spend in the most cost-effective way possible. We do this by bargaining with drug companies to keep prices down. Experienced doctors and medical staff look at how effective different medicines are across different medical conditions and help us decide what to fund.' It's a logical way of responding to a complex dilemma.

There is one obvious absentee from this list of countries: America. As a 2017 article in the *Huffington Post* stated, 'Given that the US has the most expensive healthcare in the world, with comparatively low value and outcomes compared to many other advanced countries, you would think that CEA (cost-effectiveness analysis) would be a major part of health policy in this country. Sadly, the opposite is true, and it is notably absent from the way we do things.'[15] Indeed, the US Medicare programme is legally required to pay for any drug that the Food and Drug Administration approve without any negotiation on price. However, research showed that between 2008 and 2012, the FDA approved most uses of cancer drugs without there being any evidence of survival or improved quality of life,[16] meaning zero price control for drugs that offer minimal benefit. How does that make any sense?

In the 1970s, two national organizations were established to regulate the American healthcare industry: the Office of Technology Assessment and the National Center for Health Care Technology. However, each of them was abolished following a backlash from powerful vested interests, especially the medical device industry and some medical professional organizations.

The most promising recent development has been the Institute for Clinical and Economic Review (ICER), an independent research organization that was founded in 2006 to objectively evaluate the value of prescription drugs, medical tests and other healthcare innovations. Such work is desperately needed – after all, most Americans have no idea how much it costs to develop a drug and they have no way of knowing if a new drug works better than any existing competitors or how much other consumers are paying for the same products. Once the lobbying power of the pharmaceutical industry over many politicians is added to the mix, this is a recipe for a rip-off. Patients deserve better.

Today, the drug assessment reports of the ICER include an analysis of how well each new drug works, the economic value of each treatment and other elements that are important to patients and their families. They use this analysis to establish a 'value-based price benchmark' that indicates how each drug should be priced in order to reflect long-term improved patient outcomes. ICER's reports also evaluate the potential short-term budgetary impact of new drugs, alerting policymakers to situations when short-term costs may strain budgets and restrict access.

Although it has no statutory role, around 65 per cent of American payers use ICER's reports as part of their formulary decisions.[17] Its influence will likely grow, which could be hugely beneficial for patients, as the following example of the first drug that it recommended a price for demonstrates.

In 2014, the pharmaceutical company Gilead Sciences introduced a new treatment for hepatitis C called Sovaldi, which challenged healthcare systems around the world because of its immense cost.

VALUING A LIFE

Hepatitis C is a virus that can infect the liver, and which, if left untreated, can cause life-threatening damage. Around 71 million people around the world currently have the condition. Treatment with Sovaldi comprised a twelve-week course of tablets that claimed to cure the infection. It was also extraordinarily expensive, at $1,000 per tablet – or $84,000 for a full course.

A subsequent drug called Harvoni, also developed by Gilead, had a cost of $94,500. This was even more effective, with a cure rate of between 95 and 99 per cent. If you only had to treat the occasional patient with this drug, it would clearly be regarded as good value; the challenge came from having to pay such a high price for the large number of people who needed it. After all, there are 3.3 million people in the US with hepatitis C, and it would cost insurers and Medicare $277 billion to cure them all. There was no way the country's free-market healthcare system could ensure that everyone who needed the drug would get it, so ICER stated that Gilead would have to cut the price of Harvoni by between one half and two-thirds, even though they had concluded that its price was cost-effective by traditional standards.[18] The next year, following intense pressure, Gilead reduced the price by 46 per cent. Although the emergence of alternative therapies in 2015 and 2016 had played a role in triggering the lower price, this price reduction was stunning – but it was absolutely necessary. It would, of course, be far preferable if users and prescribers could understand how drug prices are decided, but Big Pharma chooses to keep us in the dark.

Despite some success, costs are increasing more quickly than the funds available to pay for them – and the problem is not going away. In an article in the *New York Times*, Fiona Scott Morton, an economist at the Yale School of Management, was quoted as saying, 'The main reason we do not have a NICE-like system in the US is that drug manufacturers lose when insurers know which drug is most cost-effective. It is in Pharma's interest to protect their profits and lobby vigorously against any government body that would reveal which drugs have the highest value.'[19]

In the same article, Nicholas Bagley, a professor of law at the University of Michigan, asserted that 'If we stopped covering drugs that are 1 per cent better but 1,000 per cent more expensive, drug manufacturers would steer their research investments toward more effective drugs.' The lobbying of the pharmaceutical industry has clearly been quite extraordinarily effective at keeping prices high.

Occasionally, a logical, value-driven approach will appear. For instance, in 2012, Peter Bach and his colleagues from Memorial Sloan Kettering Cancer Center wrote a *New York Times* editorial headlined 'In Cancer Care, Cost Matters'.[20] It began powerfully: 'We recently made a decision that should have been a no-brainer: we are not going to give a phenomenally expensive new cancer drug to our patients.' Having compared the efficacy and cost of two anti-cancer agents, Zaltrap and Avastin, in the treatment of metastatic colorectal cancer and noted that Zaltrap had similar efficacy but was twice the cost of Avastin, they decided to exclude it from their hospital pharmacy. Within a week, the company producing Zaltrap had reduced its price by 50 per cent. If you've ever wanted evidence about the 'let's see what we can get away with' approach often used in drug pricing, isn't it fascinating that the company could set a price for Zaltrap and within a few weeks decide to settle for half?

Bach and his colleagues have subsequently developed DrugAbacus, an online calculator of value-based prices. Users can model prices for cancer drugs based on various factors including clinical efficacy, safety and toxicity, the value placed on a year of life and the value of innovation. The tool allows users to compare the generated values with the prices of existing drugs and has shown that between 80 and 85 per cent of cancer drugs in the United States are overpriced. Will this be a stimulus for much-needed reform?

One encouraging development in the US is what has been called 'value-based insurance design', whereby an insurer or public programme can examine the cost-effectiveness of a drug to determine how generously it could be paid for. At a lower price, insurers are prepared to offer easier access, and sales may well increase as a result.

According to the *New York Times*, a cholesterol medication called Praluent was originally priced at $14,000 per year, until ICER estimated that a cost-effective price for high-risk patients would be $8,000. So, in exchange for more favourable coverage by Express Scripts, which manages the drug benefits of 85 million people, the price was lowered. More patients will now have access to it and it will cost less per patient – what's not to like? However, we should be aware that if a similar value-based methodology were applied to existing very cheap drugs like aspirin, their price might increase dramatically. These issues are never quite as clear-cut as they seem.

The simple fact is that as funds are never infinite, difficult funding decisions are inevitable. Different patient groups will always be competing for resources and care, and QALYs at least help make decisions about the use of resources explicit and logical.

While the use of QALY scores has been criticized because of an implication that some patients will be refused treatment for the sake of others, such choices have always been made. In a debate in the House of Commons about the role played by NICE, a politician said, 'QALYs, and everything else, mean nothing to people on the street,' before going on to demand an approach based on 'fairness'. But how do you define fairness? How do you ensure that you aren't just listening to the loudest voices? When it comes to the cost of treatment, surely it is better to rely on facts than emotion?

CHAPTER 6

Better than Cure

It is such an obvious idea that it has become a cliché. The phrase 'prevention is better than cure' has been commonplace since the seventeenth century, while a version of it has been traced as far back as 1240. Surely an idea that has been around for so long must have some basis in reality? Well, yes and no. The truth is that planning and delivering prevention requires as much critical thinking and analysis as any other aspect of medicine – it should not be given automatic blanket approval.

Prevention is about helping people to stay healthy, happy and independent for as long as possible. It means stopping problems before they arise rather than treating people when they become ill. It feels entirely logical to believe that if we could manage people's health more effectively, the ever-increasing pressure on our healthcare systems would ease. A 2017 review of the cost-effectiveness of public health measures showed that 'for every £1 invested in public health, £14 will subsequently be returned to the wider health and social care economy'.[1] The benefits of preventative medicine have rarely been more obvious than during the coronavirus pandemic; the vaccination programme has exemplified the advantages of preventing disease rather than waiting to treat it.

The United Kingdom has long been an international leader in preventative medicine. In 1796, Edward Jenner developed the first smallpox vaccine. In 1854, John Snow identified the link between contaminated water and cholera by using what we now would think of as data analytics. In the 1950s, British scientists built the evidence base to establish the link between smoking and cancer. However, while exciting developments in genomics may revolutionize our ability to use preventative medicine in the treatment of some conditions, many major healthcare problems are complex, societal and extraordinarily challenging. The ways to tackle issues such as obesity, drug and alcohol abuse, dementia and mental illness are far less clear-cut than some people believe.

Action is what really matters. In 2018, the UK government said: 'We need to see a greater investment in prevention – to support people to live longer, healthier and more independent lives, and help to guarantee our health and social care services for the long term.'[2] While such words are welcome, they don't cost anything; it is noticeable that when budgets are stretched and costs need to be cut, prevention often loses out. Despite their supportive rhetoric, in December 2018 the UK government announced that public health budgets were to be slashed by £85 million in 2019–20.[3]

Analysis by the influential UK health charity the Health Foundation highlighted a £900 million real-term reduction in funding between 2014–15 and 2019–20, while the public health grant had fallen by 25 per cent per person since 2014–15. Their report said:

> Worryingly, these funding cuts come at a time when life expectancy improvements are stalling and inequalities are widening, and they have so far failed to protect the areas in greatest need. Increasing spending for the NHS while cutting funding for services that impact health is a false

economy. If the government is serious about delivering on its prevention vision, this will have to be matched with adequate funding for the things that maintain and improve people's health – not just the healthcare services that treat people when they become unwell.[4]

It's not just in the UK that public health is under-resourced. In her book *Betrayal of Trust*, the science journalist Laurie Garrett described how a series of major public health failures – including plague in India and Ebola in Zaire – contributed to what she called the collapse of global public health.[5] She accused the world's governments of failing to protect the health of the most vulnerable. Public health and prevention may not be glamorous, but they are critically important – as the coronavirus epidemic has illustrated.

What exactly we mean by 'prevention' is worth some clarification. Traditionally, there are said to be three main types of prevention: primary prevention – trying to prevent yourself from getting a disease; secondary prevention – trying to detect a disease early; and tertiary prevention – trying to reduce the symptoms of a disease you already have.

Primary prevention
Good examples of primary prevention include legislation to ban or control the use of hazardous products like asbestos, encouraging or requiring safe practices, such as the use of seatbelts, education about beneficial habits, such as healthy eating, and immunization against infectious diseases. For those who argue that people should be allowed to take whatever risks they choose, one could logically agree, provided that they understand the risks they are taking and

as long as someone else doesn't have to bear the cost of their choices when things go wrong.

Most people now understand, for instance, the logic behind the use of motorcycle crash helmets. According to the Police Foundation, 19,297 motorcyclists were injured in reported road accidents in the UK in 2016, of whom 319 were killed and 5,553 were seriously injured. According to the National Center for Statistics and Analysis, an office of the National Highway Traffic Safety Administration, 5,286 motorcyclists were killed on US roadways in 2016, a 5.1 per cent increase on the previous year.[6]

I will never forget the image of a driver's brain lying on the road, separated from the skull, when I attended one such accident – the benefits of wearing a crash helmet are clear. But why should this be a matter of legislation rather than individual responsibility?

Analysis of the costs shows that initial hospitalization and emergency treatment accounts for only 67 per cent of the total medical costs in motorcycle accident victims. In the US, additional costs include hospital readmissions, professional fees, ambulatory care services, rehabilitation and long-term nursing home care; medical and productivity savings from helmet use are estimated to be $1,316,469 per fatality, $186,434 per serious injury and $8,166 per minor injury.[7] And that's not even the end of it, because the public must also pay higher insurance rates and increased taxes.[8] In a single year, the total economic cost of motorcycle-related crashes was calculated to be more than $12.8 billion in the US alone.[9]

A further important consideration in this major American public health issue is that the cost of medical care for motorcycle crash patients is largely paid for by public money.[10] Non-helmeted motorcyclists are more likely to be covered by government-funded health insurance or to have no health insurance at all than helmeted motorcyclists.[11] Surely that makes this a matter for society rather than just a question of individual choice?

Despite this, in 2015 an Australian senate inquiry into 'nanny state' laws heard that the requirement to wear a helmet is 'bordering on ridiculousness'.[12] Although every new public health measure tends to receive the same response from the right-wing media, the debate is far from over. In the US, just nineteen states have legislation that requires all riders to wear a helmet – in many others, this is left to individual choice for riders over the age of twenty-one. As one motorcycling website explained: 'Without a national law saying that helmets are or are not required, we've ended up with a seemingly random set of laws that are different in whatever state you're in. If you wear a helmet you're always covered (literally and figuratively).'[13] Government policy is clearly not always logical.

The anti-vax campaign
Most of the measures I've mentioned so far are generally accepted to be beneficial, but there is one that is widely disputed by a small subsection of society: vaccination. I can vividly recall treating a child in Birmingham Children's Hospital many years ago who was suffering from a complication of measles known as subacute sclerosing panencephalitis that would ultimately prove fatal. When people say that measles is a trivial condition that doesn't require immunization, I would suggest they meet that poor child's heartbroken family.

Campaigners who oppose vaccination cause a great deal of distrust and immense damage, but dealing with them is far from straightforward. For instance, many parents who resist vaccination for their children are labelled as uninformed or stupid, but this is frequently not the case. They can, in fact, be extremely intelligent and well informed, but they suffer from being exposed to information that is misleading and of a poor quality.

Before the coronavirus pandemic reminded us of the critical importance of expertise – after all, no one would wish to be cared for in an intensive care unit by an amateur – there was an increasing tendency in many Western countries to dismiss experts as irrelevant. While America was led by Donald Trump, it seemed like almost every fact was contestable. Prior to the UK referendum on EU membership in 2016, the cabinet minister Michael Gove famously suggested, 'People in this country have had enough of experts.' We have now reached a point where a highly intelligent parent could spend a few hours reading page after page of anti-vaccination 'evidence' on the internet and believe that the matter is still under dispute; furthermore, they might believe that their assessment of the matter is more valid than the cumulative hours of study and experience by the overwhelming majority of medical professionals.

While this is to some extent understandable, in other ways it is mysterious. If our laptop or smartphone were to malfunction, very few of us would consider dismantling the device in an attempt to repair it – we know that repairing such electronic wizardry requires genuine expertise. So why do so many people believe that they are sufficiently equipped to analyse complex statistical data in clinical trials? For those who scoff that 'you can prove anything with statistics', the answer is, 'That might be true, but only to those people who don't understand them.'

The tendency to dismiss expertise is compounded by a desperate media desire for 'balance'. On a topic like the safety of immunization, a radio broadcast will typically pit an expert (who might represent hundreds of thousands of clinical experts) against a parent who holds contrary and highly personal opinions, with one argument inevitably being much more emotional than the other. Emotions tend to win arguments, but that doesn't mean the truth has been exposed.

For many years after the Second World War, science and rationality seemed to be winning the day, but aspects of postmodernism subsequently suggested that there is no such thing as an objective truth. In an age when politicians regularly cast doubt on truth and expertise, it is hardly surprising that our ability to trust is disrupted. Scientists such as Andrew Wakefield, the discredited author of 'research' that claimed to link the MMR vaccine with autism, first sow seeds of doubt; others then join the bandwagon, and every subsequent attempt to clarify tends to be met with cynicism. Even though Wakefield was struck off by the General Medical Council in the UK, with his work denounced as fraudulent and countless other researchers disproving his theories, he still has fervent supporters. The question of how the public regain trust in those with genuine independent expertise might be one of the most important issues of our times. True evidence-backed expertise lies behind much prevention, and this will be key to our individual and collective futures.

However, while primary prevention might be a logical and cheap solution to many issues in healthcare, it can risk ignoring the complexity of human nature. For instance, it has been estimated that 38 per cent of all premature deaths in the United States are attributable to just four health behaviours: smoking, unhealthy diet, a lack of physical activity and problem drinking.[14] But if such issues could be addressed easily, society would already have benefited immensely.

Secondary and Tertiary prevention
Rather than preventing a disease or injury from occurring in the first place, secondary prevention aims to reduce the impact of

something that has already occurred – by detecting it as early as possible and treating it in order to slow its progress. It also involves encouraging people to develop strategies that prevent recurrence and implementing programmes to return patients to good health, thereby preventing long-term problems. Examples include regular screening tests to detect disease in its earliest stages – for instance, mammograms to detect breast cancer – and screening for high blood pressure or sexually transmitted diseases such as chlamydia.

Tertiary prevention, meanwhile, aims to reduce the impact of an ongoing illness or injury, in order to improve a patient's quality of life and life expectancy. Examples include cardiac or stroke rehabilitation programmes, and long-term-condition management programmes for diabetes, arthritis or depression.

A publication by the Institute for Work and Health in Canada[15] used the example of a public health problem near a swimming hole to illustrate how these three types of prevention are different. One summer, swimmers start to develop persistent rashes, which seem to be the result of some form of chemical irritant. The exercise requires you – as mayor of this community – to take action. What might you do?

Primary prevention would require you to approach the company upstream that is discharging chemicals into the river and make it stop. Secondary prevention might involve asking lifeguards to check swimmers as they get out of the river for signs of a rash that can be treated right away – you may not be preventing the rashes, but treating them early would reduce their impact. Finally, tertiary prevention neither prevents the rashes nor deals with them right away, but involves helping people to live with them as best as possible – perhaps by setting up support groups.

As this publication concluded, many health problems require a combination of primary, secondary and tertiary interventions to achieve a meaningful degree of prevention and protection. And as this example shows, the further 'upstream' one is from a negative health outcome, the more likely it is that intervention will be effective. Preventing obesity is much more effective than tackling it once it has developed. Stopping people from smoking in the first place is much more effective than trying to wean them off nicotine. And handwashing is much more effective than treating infections after they have occurred.

Prevention, when applied appropriately, can be the most valuable, effective and cost-effective form of healthcare for both individuals and communities. To use another watery analogy, I've often heard traditional healthcare compared to the act of trying to rescue drowning people from a fast-flowing river. While the effort is courageous and to be applauded, we might more usefully follow the words of Archbishop Desmond Tutu: 'There comes a point where we need to stop just pulling people out of the river. We need to go upstream and find out why they're falling in.'

The heroic work of the fire service offers another good analogy: it is infinitely preferable to take matches away from arsonists or to ensure that all houses are fitted with a smoke alarm rather than waiting for fires to start and then rushing to put them out. However, there is no glamour in prevention – after all, who would consider dressing up as a public health official for a fancy dress party? Fire fighters are, quite rightly, regarded as heroes, but who brings the greatest overall benefit?

Similarly, it is clear that addressing any possible causes of ill health and thereby preventing sickness and disease is infinitely preferable to simply waiting for disease to strike. But despite this, there are many reasons why prevention rarely becomes a priority for spending or action.

The peril of not being glamorous

A while ago, I met with a senior UK politician. A new cardiac unit had been opened in his constituency and he was waxing lyrical about the advantages it would bring to the local population. He was, of course, absolutely right. He told me about a friend of his who had recently suffered a heart attack and been admitted to this new unit. Within a matter of hours, the man had been assessed, treated and had a coronary artery stent inserted. Within days, he was out of hospital, with a prescription for exercise at the gym. In the past, heart attack patients were typically not even admitted to hospital; the development of coronary care units, clot-busting drugs and new invasive procedures have completely changed the game.

I agreed with the politician that the unit was a stunning development that offered fantastic care, but then I asked him a question: would he prefer a heart attack to be treated rapidly and effectively, or to not have had one in the first place?

The way he looked at me quizzically made it all too clear that he thought it was a stupid question, but it illustrates one of the key challenges for any healthcare system. Do you invest in prevention? Is it better to set up an effective system that ensures that people's blood pressure is kept under control and that addresses smoking and high cholesterol, thereby preventing many heart attacks from occurring – or should you focus on providing the high-tech kit for treating heart attacks when they happen? Most countries appear to prioritize treatment – at least if we judge by their budgetary choices. You may think the answer to this question is obvious, but plenty of people will think the same about the opposite choice. So what is to be done?

SIDE EFFECTS

Imagine, for a moment, that you receive a request from a newly independent country appointing you to devise a healthcare system, with a completely free hand to design it as you wish. It is hard to believe that anyone would aim to do anything other than improve their population's health outcomes and reduce inequalities – after all, what could be more important? With this in mind, it is mystifying that so many countries appear to want their healthcare systems to do the very opposite. Why do some countries have hugely expensive MRI scanners and treatment units while lacking guaranteed quality primary care? How can it be possible to offer heart transplantation but not guarantee clean drinking water and basic hygiene? How are these priorities chosen?

A few years ago, I was privileged to address a session at the World Health Assembly in Geneva on this very issue.[16] I began by asking a few simple questions: 'How are your prioritization decisions made? Does the search for good news stories and photo opportunities trump basic front-line care? Do your populations understand this – and more importantly, do the health ministers and their civil servants?' Sadly, one suspects that they frequently do not, and the answer probably lies in our news headlines.

For good or for ill, it is individual cases that lead to headline stories. Someone who has a dramatic and effective therapy is a strong good news story, while the story of someone who fails to receive effective therapy is powerful in a different way. But tens of thousands of people *not* becoming ill isn't a story at all. If someone is prevented from having a heart attack, in all likelihood they won't even be aware of the fact.

You may have narrowly avoided a major medical catastrophe, but you will most probably have absolutely no knowledge of it. Maybe your doctor advised you to make a change to your lifestyle. Maybe you had an immunization. Maybe you managed to keep your weight down and your blood pressure stayed at an optimum level. You can't feel relieved or grateful as nothing happened, but the illness and associated problems that you avoided would have radically altered your life. It's a difficult idea to get your head around, isn't it?

Human stories frequently tend to relate to problems, but they very rarely deal with prevention. Nevertheless, I suspect that the most effective things I did in the course of my career resulted in nothing happening. There's no glamour in prevention – following up on hundreds of patients with high blood pressure seems infinitely less exciting than saving the lives of people who have been taken ill. And when doctors talk among themselves about their work, they inevitably focus on diagnosis and cure. They almost never talk about prevention, other than to moan about how boring and work-intensive it can be. However, while it's less exciting and frequently tedious, it's infinitely preferable.

My long-held belief is that one of the major drivers of global health policy is a fear of negative health stories in the media. A personal story that triggers a media scandal will generally result in action – politicians have to be seen to be effectual – but this completely ignores the key role of prevention, of straightforward, evidence-based healthcare. If an action doesn't deliver positive headlines while allowing decision-makers to take the credit, it becomes far less attractive. After all, what's the point – from a purely political perspective – in taking an action that has the potential to save thousands of lives if no one is going to notice? Or even worse – if a future government, potentially from a different political party, might take the credit. I feel like I'm probably being too cynical, but I don't know how else to understand why some activities are prioritized while others are ignored or downplayed.

Primary care

From a national policy perspective, there is no doubt that one of the least dramatic areas of healthcare is also one of the most potent. The evidence that high-quality primary care is the secret to effective healthcare is overwhelming, but most normal people don't talk about it. General practice is a key part of primary care, but it's not the whole thing. Primary care describes the first point of contact for the majority of people who need to access health services. Globally, it has been estimated that it is able to meet between 90 and 95 per cent of all health and personal social service needs. In 1978, the World Health Organization set out a broad definition of what primary care should be at their conference in Alma-Ata, Kazakhstan. The definition says primary care should:

- Be an integral part of the whole health system, as well as the wider social and economic development of the community
- Ensure greater community participation
- Act as the first point of contact for health and social needs
- Be a process that also provides ongoing care
- Be scientifically sound, practical and affordable

I spent most of my career in general practice, but I can assure you that my enthusiasm is not driven simply by my own experience. Both the World Health Organization and the World Bank have reached the same conclusion and are involved in the Primary Health Care Performance Initiative, whose website states: 'We strive to help create a world where strong primary healthcare is the reality, not the exception, for every person, family and community. PHCPI was built on the belief that primary healthcare is the cornerstone of sustainable development.'[17] A declaration by G7 ministers in 2019 said much the same thing.[18]

According to a paper in the *British Medical Journal* in June 2007: 'Primary care systems seem to offer important advantages within healthcare systems in terms of cost containment and the health of the population. Those that focus on secondary care offer the least in terms of benefits to the population overall.'[19] This is a pretty consistent global view, but the rhetoric tends not to be followed by action.

In the autumn of 2019, the World Health Organization produced a report that coincided with a major meeting on universal health coverage.[20] At a press conference to announce it, Peter Salama, head of the universal health coverage division at the WHO, stated that global health services had improved, with the gains primarily attributable to increased access to treatment for infectious diseases and improvements in access to reproductive, maternal and child health services.[21] The report recommended that every country should 'immediately allocate or re-allocate at least an additional 1 per cent of gross domestic product to primary healthcare'.

Professor Barbara Starfield from Johns Hopkins University in Baltimore was one of the most respected researchers in the area of healthcare delivery.[22] Her work highlighted the remarkable benefits that accrue when healthcare systems focus on primary care: better health outcomes, higher life expectancy, higher rates of satisfaction with healthcare, lower healthcare costs and lower medication use. Those seem to me to be exactly the outcomes anyone would wish for – indeed, one might wonder what else would matter to the leaders of a healthcare system. It has been clearly demonstrated that if health systems are based on effective primary care with highly trained generalist physicians practising in the community, they provide more cost-effective and clinically effective care.[23]

However, despite its effectiveness, there is little glamour in primary care. There are no newspaper stories unless something has gone wrong, generally to do with access. In the United Kingdom, public pronouncements by politicians about education and health almost always deploy the same shorthand phrase – 'schools and hospitals' – for use in headlines.[24] Perhaps this isn't entirely surprising – after all, about 80 per cent of any healthcare budget goes into secondary care, and hospitals are where the potential for dramatic glory is concentrated.

Mercifully, the NHS in England has eventually recognized the importance of primary care, along with the fact that failing to invest in it is a false economy. The NHS Long Term Plan, announced in 2019, focused on the importance of primary care,[25] but this followed years of significant underinvestment. In very many other countries, the situation is similar; primary care remains the poor relation of healthcare.

You may be beginning to wonder what any of this has to do with prevention, but I strongly suspect that one of the key reasons for the profound effect quality general practice has on healthcare systems is related to it. If a family GP offers advice and treatment that prevents a heart attack, nothing appears to happen. The individual might lose weight, allowing their blood pressure to fall. Maybe they will change their diet or start taking medication. And at the end of all this, nothing happens. If you're looking for a dramatic outcome, there's not so much as a sniff of one. But if someone has a heart attack and is saved by an ambulance crew that arrives at full tilt with lights and sirens blaring, followed by precise and expert care delivered by a skilful hospital doctor with impressive technical support, there *is* a dramatic story. In my career as a doctor, I can't remember receiving a single letter of thanks from a patient in whom I had prevented disaster – but how could I have done? After all, no one can ever know what *didn't happen* to them.

It may be hard for politicians – such as the MP I mentioned meeting earlier – to see that something not happening is better than a dramatic success, but I am certain that you would infinitely prefer not to have a heart attack than to be successfully resuscitated after one. A 2019 study showed that deaths from heart disease in the US were strongly linked with the available provision of primary care doctors.[26] Each ten additional primary care physicians per 100,000 people were shown to be associated with a 51.5-day increase in life expectancy, as well as declines of up to 1.4 per cent in mortality rates from common causes like cancer, heart disease and respiratory disorders. Those are big numbers.

The lead author, Dr Sanjay Basu of Stanford University, said of the study: 'Greater supply of primary care physicians appeared to increase the chances that a person would be treated for cardiovascular disease risk factors like high blood pressure or high cholesterol, or caught early for major cancers like breast cancer or colon cancer.'[27]

Despite all this evidence for the importance of primary care, the headcount of hospital medical staff in the UK grew from 87,000 to 119,000 between 2004 and 2018 – a 37 per cent increase – and within that figure, the number of hospital consultants rose by 64 per cent (from 30,650 to 50,275).[28] Over the same period, the number of GPs practising in primary care fell, a pattern that has occurred around the world.

However, the impact of primary care doesn't end there: research has shown that even *hospital* mortality rates are more closely related to the number of family doctors in an area than to the number of hospital doctors. One major study demonstrated that in order to reduce hospital deaths by 5,000 per year, the NHS would either need 9,000 more hospital doctors or 2,300 more GPs.[29] This statistic makes historical workforce priorities in the UK – and I suspect in many other countries – all the more puzzling.

In the US, studies have shown that states with higher per capita numbers of primary care physicians have lower smoking rates and less obesity than states with lower numbers of doctors. Other studies have shown that areas of America with higher primary-care-to-population ratios have much lower healthcare costs than other areas. This has been demonstrated to be the case both among the elderly who live in metropolitan areas of the US and for the total population – as well as compared to other industrialized countries.

So as healthcare costs continue to rise, triggering the affordability crisis that is this book's main theme, could part of the reason be that we're focusing our activity on the dramatic rather than the effective? And why should general practice have such a major effect on the national health? There can be little doubt that keeping patients away from hospital – except when it is essential – is generally good for them.

To take the argument further still, it seems likely that the most effective way to improve a nation's health is not by simply paying more for healthcare. The evidence suggests that money would be better spent addressing issues around education, poverty and loneliness, 'the social determinants of health'.

Social determinants of health
A report entitled 'Fair Society, Healthy Lives', published in 2010 by Sir Michael Marmot, proposed an evidence-based strategy to

address the social determinants of health in the UK – the conditions in which people are born, grow, live, work and age and that lead to health inequalities.[30] The report also further emphasized the fact that most people in England don't live as long as the wealthiest do. If you aren't at the top of the social pyramid, you are more likely to suffer illness and premature death.

The report revealed that people in England's poorest neighbourhoods will die, on average, seven years earlier than people living in the richest neighbourhoods. In addition, they not only die sooner but spend, on average, seventeen more years of their lives suffering with disability. If we really care about health and the cost of providing healthcare, we should consider statistics like this in our planning.

However, the evidence has been clear for a long time – the lower one's social and economic status, the poorer one's health is likely to be. This is a finding that should be impossible to ignore, but health policy is more devoted to firefighting than to addressing such social issues. The Marmot Review concluded that health inequalities are largely preventable; not only is there a strong case for addressing them in terms of social justice – there is a pressing economic case, too.

The Covid-19 pandemic also highlighted the dramatic impact of health inequalities. Sir Michael Marmot has carried out a further study examining the pandemic's impact on health inequalities; he concluded that inequalities in social and economic conditions before the pandemic contributed to the high and unequal death toll in the UK, and that the more deprived a local authority is, the higher its mortality rate during the crisis.[31]

It is estimated that the annual cost of health inequalities in the UK is between £36 billion and £40 billion, thanks to lost taxes, welfare payments and costs to the NHS. Marmot advocates creating the conditions that allow people to take control of their own lives as a way of addressing health inequalities. Central to his review was the recognition that disadvantage starts even before birth; as a result, he recommended that the highest priority be given to his first objective: that every child be given the best possible start in life.

The UK isn't alone in suffering from these problems. As a review of the social determinants of health in the US concluded:

> Despite the overall health improvement, significant social disparities remain in a number of health indicators, most notably in life expectancy and infant mortality. Marked disparities in various health outcomes indicate the underlying significance of social determinants in disease prevention and health promotion and necessitate systematic and continued monitoring of health inequalities according to social factors.[32]

Similar health inequalities exist in Australia. As the Australian Institute of Health and Welfare reported in 2018:

> Action on the social determinants of health is an appropriate way to tackle unfair and avoidable health inequalities. One study estimates that if action were taken on social determinants – and the health gaps between the most and least disadvantaged closed – 0.5 million Australians could be spared chronic illness, $2.3 billion in annual hospital costs could be saved and

Pharmaceutical Benefit Scheme prescription numbers cut by 5.3 million.[33]

In 2019, the Canadian government stated:

> Reducing health inequalities means helping to give everyone the same opportunities to be healthy, no matter who they are or where they live. We are working in a number of ways to reduce health inequalities and address the social determinants of health.[34]

I could go on listing countries and their statistics, but the simple fact is that this issue exists everywhere. There is little doubt that if you want to improve the health of a nation, you will achieve better results if you invest in housing and education, along with addressing the various other social factors that dramatically impact on health.

At the same time, no nation could ever abandon the provision of health services and focus on these social inequalities – even if the results achieved were much better. Sickness and disease will always happen to individuals; however effective prevention might be and however logical it might be to focus on the social determinants of health, governments simply cannot ignore healthcare provision. It might theoretically be possible to improve the quality of health through massively increasing spending on the social determinants of health, but citizens will continue to become ill with cancer, heart disease, mental health problems and an endless number of other conditions.

While no government or healthcare system could ever say, 'We've spent everything on prevention – there's nothing left for treatment,' the problem is that the opposite does sometimes happen – when times are tough, the prevention budget is generally cut. I can understand why today's crises get the lion's share of funding, but it is also breathtakingly short-sighted – another case where healthcare decision-making results from short-term budgeting rather than long-term planning.

Of course, prevention can only go so far. There is no escaping the fact that we will all eventually die, so healthcare has to focus on improving quality of life and not just on longevity. Focusing on prevention and the social determinants of health is the right thing to do, but it will not necessarily reduce costs. In fact, it might be the modern-day equivalent of the naïve fallacy that was popular soon after the birth of the UK's National Health Service; the idea that better care would lead to a healthier population and lower costs.

CHAPTER 7

Overtreatment and Overdiagnosis

The previous chapter suggested that investment in preventative medicine might solve some of the major challenges facing our healthcare systems. If we could only spot healthcare problems early enough, we could treat them before they begin to impact significantly on patients, saving both misery and at least some of the costs that might result from a later diagnosis.

On one level, this would, of course, be right – prevention is logically better than cure. Unfortunately, however, there are aspects of preventative medicine that neither prevent disease nor reduce cost. This is particularly the case with respect to some forms of screening, which has led many clinicians to talk of the concept of 'overdiagnosis'. As the American journalist H. L. Mencken once wrote, 'For every complex problem, there is an answer that is clear, simple and wrong.'

While it is entirely logical to screen for conditions where the evidence shows real benefits, some aspects of screening are unnecessary and risk increasing anxiety without there being clear evidence of any real benefit. A key duty of any doctor since the days of Hippocrates has been 'primum non nocere' – typically translated as 'first, do no harm' – but this is far from straightforward. After all, the only way you can be sure to avoid harm is by not doing anything, which in itself can be harmful. It's quite a conundrum.

Every treatment carries a degree of risk, but not acting can be even more dangerous. There is jeopardy in operating on someone who has acute appendicitis, but you would not want your doctor to refuse to consider surgery for that reason. The risk in this case is justified – unless, of course, you have another health issue that exacerbates it. Knowing when not to operate, balancing the benefits and risks, is one of the key skills of any surgeon – it sometimes requires even more skill than the act of surgery itself.

Nevertheless, there are certain activities within medicine where the risk of harm outweighs the risk of benefit. To understand why something as benign and potentially beneficial as screening might be problematic, let us consider the entirely fictional case of the identical twins Melanie and Marjorie Evans.

Imagine that in October 2029, Melanie dies of a cancer of the tropioid bone. (There is no such bone, and no such condition, but bear with me). Her cancer had been diagnosed in October 2028, meaning that she lived for a year after it was diagnosed – a heartbreaking tragedy.

Her sister Marjorie, however, had been living in a country that encouraged regular screening of the tropioid bone. After an MRI scan in 2021 identified early signs of cancer, she underwent surgical excision and radiotherapy, surviving eight years after diagnosis. Her family were immensely grateful and campaigned tirelessly in the media for greater access to this sort of screening.

But Marjorie and Melanie died on the same day, of a condition that had probably developed at the same time. One of them was diagnosed earlier, meaning a long time between diagnosis and death. The other twin was diagnosed much later and had a shorter survival time. Which of them benefitted most from medical science? Was tropioid screening of any benefit to Marjorie, or did it just mean many years of treatment, with its accompanying side effects, and many years of worry, for no extra life? The benefits of screening are not always as straightforward as one might think.

Before I go on, however – a definition. Screening refers to a strategy used across a population to identify the presence of disease in individuals who have no symptoms. It is typically carried out on people who seem to be in good health, with the intention of reducing mortality and symptomatic disease.

I have in the past read about young women who consulted their GP after developing slight but abnormal vaginal bleeding. In some cases, their doctors refused to conduct a smear test because they were not in the appropriate age range for screening; tragically, some of these young women subsequently died and their families have since campaigned for the age of screening to be changed. But cervical cytology screening is designed to detect early changes in patients with *no signs of abnormality*. Faced with any symptom, doctors should be carrying out diagnosis, not screening.

However, not all screening is beneficial, as the story of Marjorie and Melanie showed. Some programmes cause anxiety for no benefit, while others lead to overdiagnosis and overtreatment. Some cause problems by offering false reassurance, meaning that people delay consultation when they develop symptoms – 'I can ignore that bleeding because I was screened last month and everything was fine.'

The principles of screening

To try and minimize the disadvantages and maximize the benefits of screening, in 1968 the World Health Organization published guidelines on the principles and practice of screening for disease:[1]

- The condition should be an important health problem
- There should be a treatment for the condition
- Facilities for diagnosis and treatment should be available
- There should be a latent stage of the disease
- There should be a test or examination for the condition
- The test should be acceptable to the population
- The natural history of the disease should be adequately understood
- There should be an agreed policy on whom to treat
- The total cost of finding a case should be economically balanced in relation to medical expenditure as a whole
- Case-finding should be a continuous process, not just a 'once and for all' project

Some of these may sound obvious, but they all matter. For instance, the requirement that screening should be for an important condition is crucial. It might be possible to identify conditions that are both interesting and unimportant, but the fact that science *can* do something doesn't mean that it *should*. It would be a waste of time and money to be told that something unimportant is wrong with you, as well as a likely cause of anxiety.

The requirement that there must be a treatment for the condition is equally important. Indeed, one of the key challenges in any form of screening is knowing when the potential harms outweigh the benefits, which takes us on to the complex topic of overdiagnosis.

The problem of overdiagnosis

Let's take as an example the issue of raised blood pressure, a vitally important clinical topic that raises interesting challenges. High blood pressure can clearly be dangerous, and just to complicate matters, it may not cause you any symptoms at all. You may feel totally healthy – with no headaches, nose bleeds or dizziness – and yet have blood pressure that is dangerously off the scale. I am not for one moment suggesting in what follows that all high blood pressure can be ignored.

If your blood pressure is too high, it puts extra strain on your blood vessels, heart and other organs, such as the brain, kidneys and eyes. Persistent high blood pressure can increase your risk of a number of serious and potentially life-threatening health conditions, such as heart disease and heart attacks, strokes, heart failure, peripheral arterial disease, aortic aneurysms, kidney disease and vascular dementia. That's quite a list, and so screening for the condition is recommended.

This may sound straightforward, but the challenge comes from determining when the word 'high' is appropriate. Because unlike the many clearly defined illnesses that you either do or don't have, the definition of high blood pressure keeps changing.

Blood pressure is measured using two numbers. The systolic pressure (the higher number) is the force at which your heart pumps blood around your body, while the diastolic pressure (the lower number) is the resistance to the blood flow through blood vessels. As a general guide, high blood pressure is considered to be 140/90mmHg or higher, while ideal blood pressure is usually considered to be between 90/60mmHg and 120/80mmHg.

Borderline blood pressure readings of between 120/80 mmHg and 140/90 mmHg could indicate a risk of developing pathologically defined high blood pressure, but the point at which action is taken depends on the latest research. In 2017, the American College of Cardiology and the American Heart Association stated that high blood pressure should be treated with lifestyle changes or medication at 130/80mmHg rather than 140/90mmHg.[2]

These decisions can have a massive impact. For instance, a paper in the *British Medical Journal* showed that if these guidelines were introduced in the US and China, more than half of all people aged between forty-five and seventy-five would be considered hypertensive.[3] Consider what that might mean to manufacturers of blood pressure medication. And remember that while enough people will benefit to justify such treatments, most people won't receive any benefit whatsoever. The problem here results from applying epidemiological data to individuals. On a population basis there is absolutely no doubt that treating borderline high blood pressure is beneficial. However, it is much harder to interpret these data for individuals.

As an example of the problem, reviews of the evidence have shown that when it comes to systolic blood pressure levels of around 140 to 160, and looking at just one type of treatment as an example, 122 people with no prior heart attack or stroke would need to be treated with medication for just one person to benefit.[4] Of course, not having a heart attack or stroke is a very significant benefit, but 121 of the 122 people would receive no benefit at all. The problem is that we currently can't tell which individual will benefit.

This concept of the 'number needed to treat' (or NNT) can be immensely helpful and can support individual patients who are trying to decide whether treatment is worthwhile for them. For higher blood pressures, for example, the NNT will be much lower, meaning that treatment is more likely to be personally beneficial. Only you can decide if it is worth taking a tablet that may or may not help you, and by knowing the NNT you are in a much better position to weigh up your personal view. Prescribing without first discussing or sharing this information is a long way from being ideal practice – hopefully the provision of the NNT will become a standard part of good medical practice.

Many doctors worry that medicine might have unwittingly become the delivery arm of the pharmaceutical industry. While the cost of treating huge numbers of patients to prevent a small number of serious incidents can be justified, there is concern that it represents the overmedicalization of society. If most of the population were prescribed pharmaceuticals to reduce their risk of heart disease, would this be a good thing? The answer is not clear-cut, but society is drifting towards it without fully debating the issues.

Anxieties about overtreatment stem not just from an unease about turning healthy people into 'patients' but from an underlying suspicion about the pharmaceutical industry. Addressing such concerns requires complete transparency about the process when treatment guidelines are drawn up and – just as importantly – for the issues to be shared with the patient. After all, whose body is it anyway?

I should stress that anxiety about overdiagnosis is not restricted to conditions like high blood pressure. Two further examples are the point at which depression is treated and the existence of prediabetes.

Depression is a very real and serious medical condition, as important as cancer or heart disease. While not every suicide is linked to depression, most cases are, and in 2017 there were 6,213 suicides in the UK and Ireland, with men about three times more likely to kill themselves than women. According to the Centers for Disease Control and Prevention, suicide claimed the lives of over 47,000 Americans in one recent year, making it the second leading cause of death among individuals between the age of ten and thirty-four, and the tenth leading cause of death overall. In the

UK, the suicide rate is highest among people aged between forty-five and fifty-nine, at 27.1 per 100,000 men and 9.2 per 100,000 women.[5] These are horrifying statistics, each one representing a tragic individual case.

Depression needs to be treated seriously, but there is no clear dividing line – a simple blood test, for instance – that distinguishes unhappiness from depression. The technical term for an important and dangerous condition is the same as the word used to describe a mood, which adds to a wealth of misunderstandings and prejudice.

In times of societal turmoil, people may present more frequently to doctors with symptoms of unhappiness, and – sometimes as a result of the unavailability of more appropriate therapies – many are prescribed anti-depressant drugs. Being on such medication does not guarantee a correct diagnosis. Indeed, as a paper in the *British Medical Journal* stated, 'Depression is now more likely to be overdiagnosed than underdiagnosed in primary care. Rates of prescribing of anti-depressant medication doubled in the UK between 1998 and 2010, and in the US 11 per cent of the population aged over eleven now takes an anti-depressant. People without evidence of major depressive disorder are being prescribed drug treatment.'[6] I'll return to this topic in a later chapter, but such figures are pertinent in a book about the increasing costs of healthcare.

Prediabetes is a growing global problem that is closely tied to obesity, and if undiagnosed or untreated it can develop into type 2 diabetes. Prediabetes is characterized by the presence of blood glucose levels that are higher than normal, but not high enough to be classed as diabetes. According to Diabetes UK:

OVERTREATMENT AND OVERDIAGNOSIS

The increasing number of new cases of prediabetes presents a global concern as it carries large-scale implications towards the future burden on healthcare. Between 2003 and 2011, the prevalence of prediabetes in England alone more than tripled, with 35.3 per cent of the adult population, or one in every three people, having prediabetes. [7,8]

This is often reported as a medical emergency, a massive challenge for healthcare systems in every country in the world. However, an article in the *British Medical Journal* warned that changes in the way in which the condition is diagnosed risks unnecessary diagnoses:

> Aldous Huxley wrote that 'Medical science has made such tremendous progress that there is hardly a healthy human left.' Changes to the American Diabetes Association guidance on the diagnosis of prediabetes in 2010 make this statement even more true. If implemented globally the guidance could create a potential epidemic, with over half of Chinese adults, for example, having prediabetes, a national burden of around 493 million people.[9]

Knowing how to interpret such data is of critical importance. As was pointed out by the *BMJ*, it is a leap of faith to believe that the treatment of people in newly defined categories will improve morbidity and mortality rates, and overdiagnosis risks significant harm. If over half the population is defined as 'sick', what is normal? Can the majority of any group really be defined as abnormal – and if they are, is the problem with the definition or the people? If this is the future we want to head towards, what will the implications be?

Imagine how you might react if analysis of insurance data in the future showed that people of a particular height had a much longer life expectancy than those who were taller or shorter. If your height was different from the optimum, would that make you abnormal or unwell? What are the implications of such an analysis?

After all, being labelled as prediabetic can bring problems with self-image, insurance and employment, as well as the burdens of healthcare costs and drug side effects. Perhaps the solution to issues that have such a massive societal impact is to address them at a population level rather than medicalizing individuals. The prime cause of such widespread obesity is clearly dietary, but tackling big businesses tends to be far harder than devolving the problem to individuals. Even where medication might not be the most logical or effective way forward, governments seem happy for these issues to be dealt with by medicine and pharmacology, causing the cost of healthcare to escalate further.

When they are diagnosing all these conditions, clinicians need guidance that takes into account as much validated research as possible. It is impossible for them to keep up to date with the constant torrent of new research, which means that clinical guidelines take on a greater importance.

Trusting guidelines

It is crucial that guidelines on the management of healthcare conditions can be trusted. In the past, some of them were barely disguised marketing materials paid for by the pharmaceutical industry; it was hardly surprisingly when they concluded that more drugs should be prescribed. The best guidelines are now produced following a series of international criteria called the Appraisal of Guidelines for Research and Evaluation (AGREE).[10] NICE used its own methodology, but with criteria that were closely linked. They looked at whether each guideline:

- Was based on the best evidence available
- Used expert input
- Had patient and carer involvement
- Used independent advisory committees
- Involved genuine consultation
- Underwent regular review
- Had an open and transparent process, and was tough on conflicts of interest
- Took into account social values and equity considerations

It is much easier to have faith in guidelines if their production adheres to these criteria. If someone reads a set of guidelines and says, 'It's hardly surprising that they recommended that drug – look who paid for them,' they simply won't be trusted. If they are to be of value, guidelines need to be trusted by clinicians and patients alike.

Shared decision-making
When we are dealing with long-term preventative treatments, it is crucial that patients are actively involved in their own care. Most of us would be inclined to ask our doctor to make the tough decisions for us if we were acutely ill with a life-threatening condition. But if we are dealing with preventative medicine, where taking a tablet *may* be beneficial and *may* have side effects, it is vitally important that the patient is central to any decisions that are taken. Shared

decision-making ensures that treatment is a collaborative process through which a clinician supports a patient as they reach decisions.

As described by NHS England, such a conversation brings together the clinician's expertise – treatment options, evidence, risks and benefits – with the things the patient knows best: their preferences, personal circumstances, goals, values and beliefs.[11] Such shared decision-making is appropriate in almost every situation where a 'preference-sensitive' care decision has to be made. This means any case where there is more than one reasonable course of action and the decision involves trade-offs, any case where the evidence for one option over another is unclear or where individual values are important in the decision.

To take a relatively straightforward example, a doctor should rarely, if ever, simply instruct a patient to take a statin indefinitely to prevent cardiovascular disease without full discussion – though I suspect that some doctors have taken this approach. In such cases, the decision to prescribe and take treatment is not cut and dried.

With statins, the vast majority of people who are prescribed them will receive no benefit at all, but a few will avoid heart disease or stroke. The problem here is the fact that we cannot tell in advance which group an individual may be in, though enough people get benefit from the treatment to make it cost-effective. If you take a group of one hundred people with a 10 per cent risk of developing coronary heart disease (CHD) or a stroke over the next decade, and none of them take a statin, over the next ten years ten of them would develop CHD or have a stroke. If, however, all of them take atorvastatin for the whole ten years, then in that time, on average, four of them will be saved from developing CHD or having a stroke. Six people will still develop CHD or have a stroke, while the remaining ninety people will not – but they would not have done anyway. And to complicate matters even further, some people who take statins may develop side effects.

So how does anyone decide what to do? In the UK, NICE has developed a decision aid[12] that helps the patient decide how important various aspects of the treatment are to them individually, while being informed of the likely benefits and risks. Sharing decision-making with the patient is beneficial in all manner of ways, not least in avoiding the treatment of those people for whom it is not personally appropriate. Mass medication without this step is not only wrong, it is also immensely wasteful.

I have a concern that despite the many benefits of our healthcare system, our approach to care has sometimes been paternalistic – clinicians have made the decisions, and the patients have been happy to be told what to do. In a modern system, this is no longer appropriate. There is little doubt that it results in wasteful overtreatment, with the pharmaceutical industry the primary beneficiary. Treatment does save lives, but we need much more transparency about the benefits and risks.

For many years while I practised as a family doctor, I had a number of American patients, relatives of US service personnel who lived on a nearby airbase. I couldn't help but notice that when I gave them a prescription, they would typically ask a stream of questions: 'What is this?' 'How long should I take it for?' 'What are the likely side effects?' 'How does it work?' 'When should I see you again?' When I gave the same prescription to a British patient, they would typically say nothing apart from 'Thank you, doctor.'

It concerned me that in the UK we seemed to have built up a benign paternalism that both sides of the consultation – doctor and patient – found easy and acceptable. I am firmly of the conviction that for healthcare systems to survive and thrive, patients must be more engaged in their care than used to be the case; mercifully, the tide is now changing.

Decisions about the appropriateness of different therapies are also complicated by many doctors being poor at understanding the benefits and harms of treatment. One study published in 2020 showed inaccuracies of a magnitude that were likely to meaningfully affect clinical decision-making and impede conversations with patients regarding their treatment.[13] The research concluded that a systems issue rather than a failure of individual learning was to blame – finding quantitative information about the benefits and harms of treatments is difficult and time-consuming. It rarely features explicitly in clinical guidelines, and most clinicians have neither the time nor the expertise to explore the original research on which advice is based. The issue of how clinicians should best communicate levels of risk to patients requires more research, followed by the development of effective tools for both doctors and patients. Ultimately, we may be able to combine the best available evidence with high-quality clinical judgement and patient preference. This, after all, was the original goal of evidence-based medicine, and it could go a long way towards addressing the challenges of overdiagnosis and overtreatment. And finally, all of this is complicated by the fact that patients generally overestimate the benefits, and underestimate the harms, of screening, treatment and tests.[14] True and effective shared decision-making could make a substantial and important difference.

At the start of this chapter, I wrote about the problems concerning the early diagnosis of a fictional bone cancer. If this left you unconvinced about the challenges raised by screening, the issue of breast cancer screening may feel more real. Breast screening has been around for many years, and countless women feel that they owe their lives to it. It seems so logical – after all, if we catch something early, it is much easier to treat. However, a recent conference, co-hosted by Cancer Research UK's Early Detection Centre, concluded that: 'Decades after their implementation, cancer screening programmes carry the burden of unresolved ethical issues and questionable outcomes.'[15]

The problem is that screening looks only at healthy people with no symptoms. Until we get much better at being certain which abnormalities matter, there will still be uncertainty as to whether an abnormality detected on a mammogram, for instance, is important. And because we can't be certain, some healthy women will be reassured when they shouldn't be, and some women with abnormalities will have unnecessary treatment for a condition that would never have done them any harm.

Imagine two groups, each containing 200 women aged between fifty and seventy. One is screened for breast cancer and the other isn't. Of the 200 women who are screened, 185 will never have breast cancer, while fifteen will. Of these fifteen, three will die and twelve will be treated and recover. Of the 200 women who aren't screened, 185 will never have breast cancer; of the fifteen who do develop it, four will die, eight will be treated and recover, and another three will have a cancer that will never develop, a 'carcinoma in situ' in which the abnormalities remain in the breast ducts without affecting the rest of the body. If these women are not screened, they will never know about these abnormalities, they will never need any treatment and they will not be disadvantaged in any way. If they undergo screening, since we cannot know whether lesions are carcinoma in situ or a cancer that could be fatal, they are likely to be treated – sometimes with surgery. In some cases, then, early diagnosis will be harmful – but there's no way of knowing for sure.

To sum up this complex issue, screening these 200 women will save one from breast cancer while treating three unnecessarily. And just to complicate matters, it is still not clear which group – screened or unscreened – lives longer, and we don't fully understand why this is.

All of which leaves a dilemma: if breast cancer screening saves some lives while harming others, what should we do? Professor Sir David Spiegelhalter, a world-renowned statistician, was part of a team that helped to make the leaflet that is given to breast cancer patients in England more balanced. He has written, 'In summary, for every one of the survivors who "owes her life" to screening, three other women would never have been bothered by their cancer if they had not gone to screening … Recent coverage of breast screening has noted this possibility of overdiagnosis and overtreatment: the leaflet states that each year the screening programme saves 1,300 lives, but at a cost of 4,000 women offered treatment they do not need.'[16] In an interview for *Prospect* magazine, Spiegelhalter said, 'Earlier diagnosis of a serious disease might be beneficial for patients, but this should not be a foregone conclusion.'[17]

I think this complexity has two clear messages. First, we must provide clear information that people who are invited to have screening can use to decide the right way forward. We should explain that screening programmes are fundamentally designed to improve population health, and that while some people will benefit, others may have unnecessary treatment and worry. And second, these issues reinforce the importance of expertise and evidence. Opinion – however emotive – is not enough.

Think again about the screened group of women. The twelve who were treated and survived will inevitably attribute their survival to the screening; in fact, all but one of them would be mistaken, while three of them were harmed unnecessarily. Decisions around screening programmes need real evidence, but it is hardly surprising that personal stories capture the imagination more effectively than anonymous group-level statistics.

Politicians, who are rarely experts in statistics, often compound the problem. Take the former New York mayor Rudy Giuliani. In 2007, he said, 'I had prostate cancer five, six years ago. My chance of surviving prostate cancer – and thank God I was cured of it – in the United States? Eighty-two per cent. My chance of surviving prostate cancer in England? Only 44 per cent under socialized medicine.'

If only he understood the figures. In England, deaths from prostate cancer are about 19.4 per 100,000 of the population and in the US they are about 19.5 – pretty much the same. The difference is that in the US, men tend to be diagnosed earlier, making their five-year survival rates appear better – the same scenario I used earlier about Melanie and Marjorie's cancers of the imaginary tropioid bone. But Giuliani chose to use poorly applied statistics as 'evidence' to support his political beliefs.

A report in the *Medical Journal of Australia* showed that of certain cancers identified in Australia, one in five cases would have remained harmless had they not been discovered.[18] The research examined five of the cancers that are most likely to be overdiagnosed and argued that more than 50 per cent of melanomas, 22 per cent of breast cancers and 42 per cent of prostate cancers should have been ignored. Instead, most were treated with chemotherapy or surgery, treatments which carry risks for patients. Paul Glasziou, who led the study at Bond University in Queensland, said that a sharp increase in skin cancer screening in Australia had led to huge numbers of harmless moles being removed from patients. The report concluded:

Despite the uncertainties in our estimates, the estimated rates of cancer overdiagnosis have important implications for health policy. First, rates of avoidable overdiagnosis need to be reduced to the lowest level compatible with targeted screening and appropriate investigation. We also need to examine strategies for reducing overtreatment of low-risk prostate, breast and thyroid cancers … A second, and perhaps more important implication is that health services need to be alert to new areas of overdiagnosis and to detect them early.

According to a report in *The Times* on this study, Sanchia Aranda of Cancer Council Australia pointed out that doctors do not always know which cancers pose a threat – 'not diagnosing cancer and having a woman die would be considered a bigger harm than the damage of getting a cancer diagnosis that was of a cancer that might not have harmed you'. Furthermore, if you have a lesion removed and believe it might have killed you, you will always feel grateful for such screening. This is why properly conducted studies are so critical, and why Rudy Giuliani's approach is understandable but wrong.

Issues like this matter hugely to the sustainability of any healthcare system. Early diagnosis and prevention may sometimes be a very good thing, but a blanket assertion that this will benefit our struggling systems is far from the truth.

The US Preventive Services Task Force, a body of independent experts in evidence-based medicine, strongly recommends broad-based screening for only a few conditions. Their strongest recommendations include screening for high blood pressure, HIV infection, cervical cancer, and colorectal cancer in adults aged between fifty and seventy-five. There are also areas where screening is recommended but where the potential benefit isn't as strong, and they include breast cancer screening for women aged between fifty and seventy-four in this category. Prostate cancer is listed as a 'Grade C' recommendation – the net benefit appears small and men should seek professional advice before choosing to be screened.

However, for the great majority of conditions studied by the task force, there is either insufficient evidence to recommend screening or the benefits don't seem to outweigh the harms. Nevertheless, plenty of groups promote screening to a puzzled and often fearful public. These include medical device and pharmaceutical companies, advocacy groups, hospitals and medical specialty groups that benefit from screening. Although they may have good intentions, they often have something to sell – and they are also aware that emotive stories play well in the media.

Over and over again, a major result of screening is overdiagnosis – finding conditions that don't matter, generating anxiety and using healthcare resources to pursue a cure that was not required in the first place. There are two major causes: overdetection and over-definition of disease.[19] And in each case, the result is the same: patients are labelled with diagnoses that cause them more harm than benefit.

Overdetection

Overdetection refers to the identification of abnormalities that were never going to cause harm for several reasons: they either do not progress, they progress too slowly or they resolve without treatment.[20] The increasing use of high-resolution diagnostic technologies means that the detection of lesions that some doctors describe as 'incidentalomas' is growing, and these can really matter.

Consider a patient who has had a chest CT scan for no very clear-cut reason – as an attempt to reassure an extremely anxious patient with vague chest symptoms, for example – and a small lesion is noted. Once a doctor knows about such a condition, there is an obligation to investigate further, but taking a biopsy of a chest lesion carries significant risk. In this situation, an unnecessary test may risk causing significant harm. Tests should be carried out when there is a good clear indication. Overuse is not just a cause of waste; it is a cause of potential harm.

Indeed, it is clear that the more tests a clinician orders or a patient requests, the more likely it is that a 'disease' will be diagnosed. A particularly striking example was the use of ultrasound in South Korea to investigate the thyroid gland.[21] Between 1999 and 2008, the incidence of detected and treated thyroid cancer increased more than six-fold, but 95 per cent of these cancers were small and detected through screening. Significantly, the mortality rate from thyroid cancer remained unchanged over the same period. As the authors of a paper analysing this 'epidemic' concluded, 'Concerted efforts are needed at a national level to reduce unnecessary thyroid ultrasound examinations in the asymptomatic general population.'

Even when abnormalities are detected, the best approach may not be obvious, a problem compounded by what Professor Al Mulley describes as 'preference misdiagnosis'. Most doctors aspire to excellence in diagnosing disease, but as Mulley points out, far fewer aspire to excellence in diagnosing patients' preferences.

A report for the King's Fund in the UK presented evidence in areas as diverse as benign prostate disease, abnormal uterine bleeding, coronary heart disease and back pain. It showed that when patients are fully informed, they are significantly less likely to choose surgery.[22] This wasn't just a question of persuading them not to proceed with an operation; where the evidence was clear that surgery would be beneficial, more patients were likely to choose it after they had been informed of the evidence and assisted in weighing up the risks and benefits. However, only half of patients in the UK say they were always involved in decisions regarding their care. Misdiagnosing patients' preferences may be less obvious than misdiagnosing disease, but the consequences for the patient can be just as severe.

Over-definition and disease mongering
The over-definition of disease can occur either by lowering the threshold for a risk factor or by expanding the definition of a disease to include patients with ambiguous or very mild symptoms. The example I gave earlier of how thresholds for the management of high blood pressure are changed is an example of the first of these phenomena. The benefits of lowering the blood pressure of patients with marginally raised pressure will be far fewer than can be gained from tackling the problem in people with much higher pressure.

Blanket approaches to treatment are clearly to be avoided. Rather than automatically writing out a prescription, clinicians should share the relevant information with their patients and work with them to determine the best approach. After all, overdiagnosis, far from offering any benefit, might have negative physical, psychological, social and financial consequences.

Included in the category of over-definition is the concept of 'disease mongering', which many believe has been a core strategy in marketing campaigns for conditions including hair loss, restless legs syndrome, shyness and even loneliness. The term, which describes the invention or promotion of diseases primarily to capitalize on their treatment, was first used in 1992 by the science writer Lynn

Payer.[23] While there are those, particularly in the pharmaceutical industry, who strongly dispute the concept, a report for the Policy Department of Economic and Scientific Policy of the European Parliament in 2012 said the following:

> Disease mongering is the promotion of pseudo-diseases by the pharmaceutical industry aiming at economic benefit. Medical equipment manufacturers, insurance companies, doctors or patient groups may also use it for monetary gain or influence. It has increased in parallel with society's 'medicalization' and the growth of the pharmaceutical complex. Due to massive investments in marketing and lobbying, ample use of internet and media, and the emergence of new markets, it is becoming a matter of concern, and policymakers should be aware of its perils and consequences.[24]

Professor Helen Stokes-Lampard, then chair of the Royal College of General Practitioners, added:

> Disease mongering is scaremongering and it has the potential to cause huge strain for the NHS and other healthcare systems around the world. Giving people unnecessary medical labels causes anxiety and distress and, in the worst cases, causes harm that can ruin lives. It also leads to unnecessary workload burdens in general practice and secondary care, and consumes funding that could be much better spent elsewhere on the care of patients who really need it.[25]

In Canada, it has been estimated that patients receive more than a million potentially unnecessary tests and treatments each year.[26] However, the problem of overdiagnosis may turn out to be even more serious in low- and middle-income countries.[27] In a global healthcare system that is struggling to contain costs, expanding the definition of disease to include more and more patients for minimal genuine benefit is hardly a logical way forward.

Ray Moynihan, who has conducted research into disease mongering, summed up the weirdness of our current situation in an interview for the *Atlantic* magazine:

> We seem to be living through the most extraordinary paradox: we have never been healthier, yet we seem to consider ourselves sicker and sicker than ever. Mild symptoms, inconvenience, being at low risk, ageing, human life, and death, are rapidly being medicalized.[28]

This bizarre situation may have all manner of explanations. Some of it is linked to overdiagnosis and disease mongering, which is worse in those countries where consumer advertising by the pharmaceutical industry encourages the public to consider particular emotions or minor symptoms as requiring medical treatment by pharmaceutical medicines. As a 2002 paper in the *British Medical Journal* explained, 'there's a lot of money to be made from telling healthy people they're sick'.[29]

Part of the problem is the widespread practice of 'churnalism', a pejorative term to describe the way in which under-resourced journalists reproduce press releases – in this case produced by the pharmaceutical industry. These stories are then amplified thanks to the extraordinary impact of social media. A bit more journalistic scepticism about 'wonder drugs' would not go amiss. As the *BMJ* has said, 'We suggest that health professionals, policymakers, journalists and consumers move away from reliance on corporate sponsored material about the nature or prevalence of disease.'

However, the causes of our anxiety about health that drive so much demand in our healthcare system are incredibly complex. When media stories about patients with rare and dangerous conditions describe the difficulties patients may have had getting a diagnosis – 'the doctors kept reassuring me' – it illustrates why reassurance from the medical profession is less effective now than it was in a paternalistic era of healthcare where 'doctor knew best'. A number of developments might improve this: a return to greater continuity of care, easier access to appropriate investigations, and enhanced communication training for clinicians. These are hardly short-term aspirations, but they would all bring great potential benefits.

In addition, in many countries around the world, the family doctor is the only readily available source of advice in difficult times. In the past, families tended to have multi-generational support structures; today, they are more likely to be geographically dissipated, and the support isn't there in the same way. Fewer people now go to their priest, vicar or rabbi when they are troubled – but they do go to their doctor. I know we should be honoured to have this responsibility, but the fact that everything is our business makes it increasingly difficult to know when we have succeeded.

As the old saying goes, 'To a man with a hammer, everything looks like a nail.' If someone goes to their doctor with a problem, it is hardly surprising that the doctor will tend to think in medical terms. As a doctor, I'm all too aware that we often use the medical model because it's what we know, but this does not mean that it will always be appropriate. Some of the problems get brought to us because the patient doesn't have anyone else they can turn to.

We all know about Rorschach tests, or the illustrations where we either see two elderly women or a vase depending on how we look at them. In a similar vein, I can't help but wonder if the reason that doctors find medical solutions to people's problems is simply because that's what we do. As a doctor, I was trained to use a medical model when approaching a patient with a problem – looking for a clear diagnosis and offering an appropriate treatment. Indeed, patients have almost been 'trained' to expect this and may be disappointed if their doctor doesn't use this approach. Doctors frequently worry that patients will make a complaint and resort to litigation if they are not seen to be doing everything technically possible to help. When a medical diagnostic approach is truly appropriate, doctors can make a real difference. But when we get it wrong, we risk finding a disease where there isn't one. However, as much as we might want to, moving away from this model will be challenging.

CHAPTER 8

Hearts and Minds

Which is more important, depression or cancer? This probably sounds like a completely absurd question – a bit like asking whether apples are superior to carrots, or whether Tuesday is better than wi-fi. But there is little doubt that many people – policymakers and politicians in particular – have indirectly answered this question with their actions, even if they didn't intend to. And their response has a profound effect on how our healthcare system operates.

For the past few years in England, when a family physician suspects that one of their patients might have cancer, the National Health Service prioritizes their care to the extent that all referrals should be seen by a specialist within two weeks. Time matters, and so this system should be designed to trigger immediate action to ensure effective care is offered as quickly as possible. On a personal level, I have seen this working for myself. Once my own tonsillar cancer had been initially suspected, a multi-disciplinary team swung into action. On the first day that I was seen at the hospital where I would receive all my treatment, I was assessed by two ENT surgeons, one oncologist, two specialist nurses, a dietician, a dentist, a speech and language therapist and even an audiologist to arrange a baseline test of my hearing, in order to monitor any potential adverse effects of chemotherapy. I was hugely impressed, and confident that I wasn't just receiving this treatment because I was at that time very senior in the NHS. My experience was the same as all the patients that I spoke to, which was exactly as it should be. It is also important to note that this was just before the Covid-19 pandemic, which had such a devastating impact on an already stretched healthcare system.

By contrast with my personal experience, let us remember the report that found that eight out of ten NHS trust finance directors in England agreed that funding pressures had led to longer waiting times for people in need of mental health treatment.[1] And even after patients had been able to access mental health services, cost-cutting had led to shorter courses of treatment and less contact with services. It's quite a contrast with the way the system approaches cancer.

In the US, the waiting time for patients with psychiatric emergencies is disproportionately longer than for other patients.[2] According to the American College of Emergency Physicians, three-quarters of emergency room doctors reported that they see patients who need psychiatric hospitalization at least once every shift; despite this, 83 per cent of emergency departments do not have an on-call psychiatrist.

In Canada, it has been estimated that one-fifth of the population lives with a mental illness; more than 60 per cent of them are reluctant to seek treatment for fear of being stigmatized, while the waiting times for psychotherapy are much longer than for physical conditions.[3] In Australia, the death rate for people receiving mental health treatment is almost twice as high as the general population.[4] Figures from a report by the Australian Bureau of Statistics found that the standardized rate of death for people seeking government-subsidized mental health treatment was 11.4 deaths per 1,000 people, nearly double the death rate among the general population.

In case you suspect that I might be cherry-picking countries with a poor record, a study in *World Psychiatry* looked at the World

Health Organization's World Mental Health survey, which stated:

> Worldwide, mental disorders inflict tremendous morbidity, mortality and impairment. Although the armamentarium of effective treatments keeps growing, few nations seem able or willing to pay for their widespread use.[5]

Back in England, an initiative called Improving Access to Psychological Therapies provides therapy for adults with conditions including depression, post-traumatic stress disorder and anxiety. While nine out of ten patients have an initial assessment within six weeks, treatment typically starts with the second appointment. Half of patients waited over twenty-eight days for this, with one in six waiting for more than ninety days.[6]

A report in the *Health Services Journal* found that hundreds of young people assessed as requiring specialist mental health treatment had been made to wait more than a year. Of the 11,482 young people assessed as needing specialist care, 5,648 (50 per cent) waited more than eighteen weeks. A total of 539 waited more than a year, with one child waiting nearly two and a half years. Only 1,630 young people, or 14 per cent, began treatment within four weeks.[7] Again, consider the contrast with the urgency of cancer referral. It would be absurd, unacceptable and dangerous if cancer was treated with less urgency, but waiting two and a half years for urgent mental healthcare is absurd, too.

How can these differences make sense? You might think that the answer is straightforward and based on risk – after all, cancer is a potential killer. But as I told the House of Commons Health Select Committee in 2013 when asked about a government initiative called the Cancer Drugs Fund, you are just as dead from suicide as you are from cancer. Suicide is the tenth most common cause of death in the US. In 2018, it was responsible for 6,507 deaths in the UK, where it is the most common cause of death for men aged between twenty and forty-nine. If a relative of yours were to kill himself during an episode of severe depression, you would feel just as bereaved as you would if cancer or heart disease was to blame. Death has no respect for labels.

Parity of esteem?
Whatever the rhetoric spoken by politicians, mental health problems are clearly taken less seriously than physical health problems. This has been recognized for some years; in response, campaigners have called for 'parity of esteem', meaning that mental and physical health would be given equal priority. According to the Mental Health Foundation, this would result in those with mental health problems benefitting from equal access to the most effective and safest care and treatment, equal efforts to improve the quality of care, and equal status within healthcare education, practice and outcomes. This would result in the allocation of time, effort and resources on a basis commensurate with need, in addition to equally high aspirations for service users.

Of course, it is widely recognized that physical and mental health are intrinsically linked, with poor mental health increasing the risk of physical health problems. There is also growing evidence to demonstrate the importance of inflammation in both bodily disorders and brain disorders. As Professor Edward Bullmore from the University of Cambridge has written:

> Currently, physical and mental health services are sharply segregated, reflecting a philosophical prejudice against viewing the mind and body as deeply intertwined ... In contrast, the new science of inflammation and the brain is clearly aligned with arguments for breaking down these barriers in clinical practice. More than that, though, it has the potential to transform our thinking about illness more broadly. The barrier between mind and body, for so long a dogmatic conviction, appears to be crumbling.[8]

However, the barrier is crumbling far too slowly – sadly, this 'parity of esteem' has all too often been little more than a parroted platitude. There are rare and admirable politicians who are prepared to acknowledge the issue and do something about it, but physical illness continues to trump mental health when it comes to prioritization. And the blame does not only lie with politicians and leaders – after all, it is society and the media that create an uproar if the treatment of physical illness is delayed or denied. By comparison, waiting lists for mental health issues barely cause a ripple on society's list of concerns.

I am certain that most clinicians would deny being at all prejudiced about mental health issues. The standard rhetoric is that 'it is nothing to be ashamed of' and 'no different to breaking a leg', but I am struck by what I have personally witnessed during my career. On many occasions, I have spoken at conferences of healthcare professionals about my own experience of mental health problems, and yet I cannot recall a single occasion when I have not been congratulated for being 'open and honest' about my depression. 'I thought that was really brave,' well-meaning audience members will typically say.

I am sure these same people would not have told me I was brave had I talked openly about my experience of cancer, of back pain or almost any other physical condition. The very use of the phrase discloses a level of prejudice, although most people would probably deny it. How can it be 'brave' to be open about something that is 'nothing to be ashamed of'?

It is this prejudice that I believe leads to mental health being the underfunded poor relation in comparison to our physical health. This book has been written to promote a discussion about the funding of healthcare – one of the great challenges facing communities across the world. This chapter will compare two contrasting aspects of healthcare – cardiovascular disease and depression, which we might refer to as 'hearts and minds' – and reveal some instructive and puzzling differences. I am in no way saying that one is more important than the other – I'm simply asking why most healthcare systems regard them as being so very different.

Hearts ...

Just as there are multiple forms of mental health problem, there are a multiplicity of different varieties of heart disease, from congenital heart disease to inflammation and infection, valvular disease, disorders of the heart's rhythm and congestive heart failure. However, by far the most common, and the one that gets the most publicity, is coronary heart disease.

CHD occurs when the blood supply to the heart is blocked or interrupted by a build-up of fatty substances in the coronary arteries. In those people who are susceptible, the artery walls become furred up with fatty deposits, a process known as atherosclerosis that is caused by various lifestyle factors and other conditions, such as high blood pressure and diabetes. It is extraordinarily common, and not just in the elderly. A study of post-mortems on US soldiers killed during the Vietnam War showed that 45 per cent of them had some evidence of atherosclerosis, while 5 per cent showed evidence of severe coronary atherosclerosis.[9] The average age of combat soldiers in Vietnam was just nineteen.

Every year, cardiovascular disease causes an estimated 17 million deaths, one-third of all deaths worldwide.[10] In developed countries, heart disease and stroke are the first and second leading cause of death among adults. While the situation has been improving in many places, the burden of cardiovascular disease in developing countries has increased to the extent that it causes twice as many deaths as in developed countries.

In the US, one person dies from cardiovascular disease every thirty-seven seconds. This equates to approximately 647,000 people each year – approximately a quarter of all deaths. And in addition to the massive human cost, the financial impact is huge. It has been estimated that heart disease costs the country about $219 billion each year,[11] including the cost of healthcare services, medicines and lost productivity due to death.

As a result of this carnage, the prevention of heart disease has been a focus of most Western healthcare systems for many years, with the introduction of various health checks and campaigns about diet, blood pressure, smoking and exercise. It is treated as a priority – if your doctor suspects you have heart disease, you are likely to have special investigations arranged as a matter of urgency, with the potential for medication, follow-up and support.

... And minds

If you develop depression, the healthcare system tends to act with much less urgency, but it is still a hugely important condition.

According to a paper in the *British Medical Journal,* depression is the leading cause of disability worldwide and a major contributor to the planet's disease burden.[12]

The global prevalence of depression and depressive symptoms has been increasing in recent decades.[13] According to the World Health Organization, its lifetime prevalence ranges from 20 per cent to 25 per cent in women and 7 per cent to 12 per cent in men.[14] It is also a significant determinant of quality of life and survival, accounting for approximately 50 per cent of psychiatric consultations and 12 per cent of all hospital admissions.[15]

Depression is also particularly common in patients who have other health conditions. For instance, people with rheumatoid arthritis are three times more likely to suffer from depression and chronic fatigue than the general population. A UK study showed that even though chronic fatigue affects 89 per cent of people with rheumatoid arthritis, 79 per cent of sufferers said that a healthcare professional has never tried to measure their levels of fatigue, while just under half (47 per cent) have never spoken to their specialist nurse or rheumatologist about it.[16] Moreover, studies have shown that if depression occurring with rheumatoid arthritis is not effectively addressed, the treatment for rheumatoid arthritis itself can be less effective.

It is unclear whether depression in people with rheumatoid arthritis occurs *as a result* of their physical symptoms, or if it itself is a symptom. However, I have all too often heard of rheumatoid arthritis sufferers who, on discussing their depression with their rheumatologist, are told, 'You'll need to discuss that with your family doctor or get a mental health referral.' This is an extraordinary example of a medical specialty being defined by doctor's interests rather than the patient's needs. Depression and tiredness matter more to many patients than the joint pain and swelling caused by rheumatoid arthritis and should be the equal focus of any doctor treating them. On top of this, it is clear that people who have both rheumatoid arthritis and depression typically respond better to treatment when both conditions are addressed. The persistently prejudicial split between mind and body is the cause of many problems.

The funding dilemma
The challenge facing every health system is that you can only spend money once. If your priorities are focused on physical health, there will not be enough money left to give mental health problems the attention they require. In addition, current research indicates that the correlation between mental and physical health is stronger than we previously believed. Our focus on the physical will likely prove to be short-sighted.

Where, for instance, are the preventative equivalents of regular blood pressure and cholesterol checks when it comes to mental health problems? The healthcare system tries to be proactive in its treatment of hearts, but when it comes to minds, it seems happy to wait for problems to develop.

One positive development has been the concept of 'mental health first aid', a training programme that teaches the public how they might help a person developing a mental health problem or in a mental health crisis. Like traditional first aid, it is not designed to teach people to treat or diagnose mental health problems, but to offer support until professional help is received or the crisis resolves itself.[17]

Overall, there can be little doubt that the rigid divisions between physical and mental health are increasingly seen as arbitrary, and the focus on the physical at the expense of mental health issues may eventually be regarded as illogical and prejudicial. We can only hope that the long-term allocation of healthcare budgets reflect this change in attitude, but this is unlikely to happen without public pressure. When waiting times for mental health services create the same angry headlines as excessive waits for heart disease or cancer treatments, we may see action.

CHAPTER 9

Age and Ageing

I'm a problem – or at least that's what journalists and politicians keep telling me. As a headline in the *Daily Mail* in May 2013 tactfully put it, 'Elderly Population Pushing NHS to Brink of Collapse, Says Minister'.

Over the past year or so, the claim that the ever-increasing costs and challenges facing our healthcare system are primarily the result of our 'ageing population' has become more common. I've lost track of the number of academic papers I've read and lectures I've listened to that have claimed that oldies like me are the problem. Countless news broadcasts and newspaper articles mention the phrase as if it explains everything – bizarrely, our 'ageing population' has been depicted as a thoroughly undesirable development, a source of expense and problems rather than an astonishing achievement and a remarkable potential resource. And in a book about the escalating costs of healthcare, it is not a topic that I can ignore.

Although I try to keep my emotions out of these discussions, I have to disagree with this narrative. As someone who has been fortunate enough to live to a far greater age than both my father and my brother, I think the fact that many of us are now living substantially longer than our forebears is a positive development and something to celebrate. However, I am also aware that age is not everything – quality of life and health matter, too. This idea is captured by a quote that was once attributed to Abraham Lincoln: 'It's not the years in your life that count – it's the life in your years.' In many surveys, people make it clear that they don't want to live to extreme old age if it means a long, drawn-out senescence. As the old joke goes, 'They say I'll live an extra two years if I give up smoking and drinking – I just don't want to spend them in a care home.'

Those of us who retain our health into later life have a great deal to look forward to. The neuroscientist Daniel Levitin has examined World Health Organization data from sixty countries and has shown that while happiness declines in our thirties, it picks up again when we reach the age of fifty-four, peaking at the age of eighty-two.[1] In an interview he said, 'You realize you've gotten through all these things that were stressing you out. If you make it to eighty-two, you know you've managed [and] you're OK.' Indeed, he attributes happiness in old age to people readjusting the 'too-high expectations' of their youth to 'realize that life is pretty good'.

This positive take on the ageing process, while welcome, is certainly not unique. In his practical book on ageing, *De Senectute*, Cicero stated that people write off old age for four reasons: it stops you working, it makes your body weak, it denies you pleasure and every day moves you one step closer to death. But he goes on to show why these arguments are not inevitable: 'The old retain their wits quite well, if but they exercise and practise them.' He may have been writing 2,000 years ago, but his words remain as true as ever.

Since Cicero's day, the change in global demographics has been remarkable. According to the United Nations, since 2018, people aged sixty-five or above have outnumbered children under five for the first time in history.[2] The forward projections are equally remarkable. The number of people aged over eighty in the world is expected to triple between 2019 and 2050, from 143 million to 426 million.

SIDE EFFECTS

The Office for National Statistics has projected that in fifty years' time there will be an additional 8.2 million people aged sixty-five and over in the UK – a population roughly the size of present-day London.[3] To illustrate just how far things have changed already, when King George V sent the first royal telegram to a centenarian in 1917, it was handwritten and delivered by bicycle. One hundred years later, the monarchy employs seven people to administer the programme that delivers many thousands of one-hundredth-birthday congratulatory messages. Estimates suggest around about 10,000 messages are sent every year, with this number doubling annually since the current queen came to the throne in 1953.

As we have seen elsewhere, this improvement in life expectancy is far from universal – there can be great variation within a single country, or even within a city. At a time when most people died of infectious diseases, the steady rise in life expectancy reflected an improvement in both quality and quantity of life, but things are now very different. Some people enjoy a happy and healthy old age; others match them in longevity but are burdened with multiple health problems and disabilities. As Robert Louis Stevenson wrote, 'There is only one difference between a long life and a good dinner: that, in the dinner, the sweets come last.' Not everyone is in a position to enjoy the metaphorical 'sweets' at the end of their life.

If you are a seventy-year-old man living in America today, the chance that you will die in the next year is just 2 per cent.[4] In 1940, that same probability was reached at the age of fifty-six. In the developed world today, approximately 90 per cent of people will reach their sixty-fifth birthday, with the great majority of them being in a healthy condition at that age.

Diminishing returns

However, when it comes to life expectancy, we may well have reached a point of diminishing returns. By the calculations of the popular science writer Bill Bryson, if a cure for all cancers were discovered tomorrow, it would probably add little more than three years to our overall life expectancy. Eliminating all forms of heart disease, meanwhile, would add barely five years.

The reason for this is relatively straightforward: people who die of these conditions tend to be old already. Indeed, as the paleoanthropologist Daniel Lieberman has noted, for every year of extra life that has been achieved since 1990, only ten months are likely to be healthy.[5] Nearly half of everyone aged over fifty suffers from some sort of chronic pain or disability – we have become much better at extending life, but not much better at extending its quality.

In his book *The Changing Mind*, Daniel Levitin writes about the difference between healthy and unhealthy longevity.[6] He says:

> We talk about lifespan as the length of time that one is alive. Except for cases of death by accident, most of us will die of some kind of disease, or parts will just wear out. You can think of the timeline of your lifespan as being divided into two parts: the period of time that you're generally healthy (the lifespan) and the period of time that you're sick (the disease span).

It is obviously important to minimize the disease span, but as I stressed earlier, every time a human *doesn't* die of a condition, they have the opportunity to die of something else. As a result, we have a large number of people who are living *with* long-term conditions rather than dying *from* them – but their continued existence can be a positive episode in their life rather than a negative downwards spiral.

As long ago as 1997, Hiroshi Nakajima, then the director general of the World Health Organization, said, 'Increased longevity without quality of life is an empty prize.'[7] Japan has really taken notice of this message. As the country with the highest life expectancy in the world, it is investing a great deal of time and effort into promoting healthy – rather than simply numerical – old age, and ensuring that all Japanese people benefit equally.

Meanwhile, in the UK there is a huge discrepancy in the number of healthy years lived after the age of sixty-five, depending on geographical variation in the social determinants of health. For instance, if you live in the south-east of England, you are likely to have at least eight more years of life without disability than if your home is in the north-east. The UK is a relatively small country, which makes this variation even more significant.

As a result, researchers now measure not just life expectancy, but 'healthy life expectancy', a much more important concept. After all, the actual length of one's life may disguise very different experiences. Two sisters might each live to the age of ninety-nine, but one of them might have a low quality of life from the age of sixty, with a multiplicity of disabling conditions, while the other could be active until her late eighties. These are very different qualities of life, despite having the same lifespan.

Healthy life expectancy is an estimate of the number of years lived in either 'very good' or 'good' general health, based on how individuals perceive their own health. An important study from the King's Fund has shown that while healthy life expectancy has increased in the UK, it has not done so at the same rate as life expectancy – as a result, many more years are spent in poor health.⁸ Although an English man could expect to live 79.6 years between 2015 and 2017, his average *healthy* life expectancy was only 63.4 years – he would have spent 16.2 years in 'not good' health. Similarly, in 2015–17, an English woman could expect to live 83.1 years, of which 19.4 years would have been spent in 'not good' health. Although women live an average of 3.5 years longer than men, much of that time is spent in poor health.

These figures matter. If a healthcare system is focused on the population experiencing a healthy and fulfilling life, simply looking at life expectancy is inappropriate. Deprivation is a huge factor here, too. The gap in healthy life expectancy between affluent and deprived areas is even bigger at birth – about nineteen years for both males and females. Those living in the most deprived areas spend nearly a third of their lives in poor health, while the figure is about a sixth for those in the least deprived areas. That's a rotten deal.

The evidence also shows that education makes a marked difference. By the time they reach the age of sixty, university graduates are likely to be in significantly better health than non-graduates. By the age of eighty-five, over half the graduates will still have only minimal impairment in their ability to function in a way that falls within the normal adult range.

These issues have been widely known for years. In the 1960s, a study of British civil servants showed that men in the lowest employment grades were much more likely to die prematurely than men in the highest grades. In the early 2000s, Sir Michael Marmot followed up this study with 'Whitehall II', with the aim of determining what lies behind this social gradient in death and disease.⁹

The study showed that the way in which work is organized, social influences outside work – including from early in life – and various health behaviours all contribute to the clear social gradient in health. The conclusion is inescapable: health and societal inequalities cannot be separated. Concentrating our efforts on treating the problems of old age will likely be far less effective than finding ways to improve people's earlier lives. As ever, we have reached a situation where we are constantly firefighting rather than trying to prevent the fires occurring in the first place.

However, the Japanese government seems to understand some of these issues. They have a policy called the Health Japan 21 initiative, which is designed to extend healthy life expectancy by more than the increase of overall average life expectancy.[10]

This book has so far focused on the massive challenge faced by governments in affording healthcare, and nowhere is it greater than in the rapidly expanding ageing population. In Japan, healthcare costs an average of 218,000 yen (£1,530) per person for people under the age of seventy-five, but an average of 930,000 yen (£6,525) per person for those over seventy-five.[11] The difference is clear. Nursing care expenses similarly increase with age, with the main cost driven by disability – the factors that distinguish a healthy life from an unhealthy one.

If healthy life expectancy can be increased – as the Japanese government intends – it should be possible to curb healthcare and nursing costs even as the number of elderly people rises. And the answer is not drugs, genomics, robots, AI or any other form of technology – even though all these things may have a part to play. Instead, the prime key is diet and physical activity. Hardly exciting, but massively effective.

In 2013, the second phase of the Healthy Japan 21 programme was launched. The 'Smart Life Project'[12] was a comprehensive programme aimed at encouraging a healthy lifestyle, from increasing fruit and vegetable consumption and exercise, to reducing smoking and alcohol consumption, to improving mental wellbeing and reducing stress – a departure from a previous focus on individual efforts for health to instead focus on improving public health, using funding in the most effective rather than the most obvious way.

A review by the Organization for Economic Cooperation and Development reported that Japan has also taken a broad approach to secondary prevention, with more extensive health check-ups and screenings than any other OECD country.[13] These include check-ups for infants and children, an annual check for all full-time employees, an annual stress test, a check specifically focused on chronic diseases and a series of other screenings, including periodic tests for osteoporosis, periodontal disease and hepatitis B and C.

It wasn't all praise, however – the OECD stated that there is considerable scope for Japan to re-examine the range of its health check-ups, in all likelihood streamlining the range of tests offered and shifting to ensure that a smaller number of people who are at high risk are completely covered. Nevertheless, focusing on keeping people active and well-nourished appears to be key.

While the only long-term solution to the affordability of healthcare in other countries will involve a greater focus on public health, this will come too late for the generation who are already elderly. And in any case, ageing does not drive costs on its own – it is the increasing number of health conditions and age-related impairments, along with proximity to death, that are most strongly linked to healthcare costs.[14] If health services want to address the needs of an ageing population in the most effective, caring and cost-effective way, we should move towards a preventive, generalist-led, person-centred model of care. Simply spending more money and offering ever-increasing levels of medical treatment to people who are near the end of their lives is the least logical of approaches. Nevertheless, it seems to be the one that many healthcare systems appear to favour, though I doubt this approach has been chosen consciously. It has simply evolved through all manner of pressures, expectations and fears – particularly a fear faced by many clinicians that families and relatives will complain if 'everything hasn't been done' for their loved one.

Encouragingly, in 2020 the UK Secretary of State for Health Matt Hancock gave a speech in which he addressed this issue of healthy ageing. As he said:

> For most of the seventy years the NHS has been in existence, we've focused on lifespan. This has seen extraordinary successes. Mass vaccination. The collapse in the adult smoking rate from 45 per cent in the 1970s to 14 per cent today. But as the NHS enters its eighth decade, it needs to focus more on *health span*: the number of years a person can expect to live healthily and independently. In our manifesto, we committed to an extra five healthy years by 2035. This is the primary long-term clinical goal we've set the NHS. Both parts are important: extra years and healthy years. Adding years to life, and life to years.

The difficulty comes in translating this rhetoric into effective action. Grand pronouncements by politicians rarely change attitudes and behaviour when clinicians and managers are faced with urgent, real-world problems, but hope remains. The UK's Centre for Ageing Better is a charity that aims to help people enjoy later life, working with partners across England to improve employment, housing, health and communities.

Furthermore, community action can have a truly profound impact. In Frome, a small town in the south-west of England, a 'compassionate community' scheme has helped cut local emergency hospital admissions by 17 per cent.[15]

'While emergency admissions to hospitals across Somerset have increased by 29 per cent, incurring a 21 per cent increase in costs, Frome has seen admissions fall 17 per cent, with a 21 per cent reduction in costs in 2016 to 2017 compared to 2013 and 2014,' said Dr Julian Abel, a palliative care consultant who is involved in the project. Health Connections Mendip, an organization set up at a local medical centre, compiled a directory of care providers and volunteers from health centres, local charities and other groups to help provide support to people with poor health.[16] These services ranged from attending to someone's physical and emotional needs to assisting with their shopping, walking their dog or helping them attend a confidence-boosting activity such as a local choir. These non-medical activities had a profound impact on health, and therefore on the cost of healthcare.

Of course, this exemplifies the fact that many aspects of health, and particularly among the elderly, are social and societal in origin. It is vitally important that we don't feel a need to medicalize the issue. Earlier in this book, I wrote about the attempts by pharmaceutical companies to develop a therapy for loneliness. A University of Chicago study is exploring whether the hormone pregnenolone can reduce the social anxiety that can perpetuate and worsen the feeling of loneliness.[17] Such an approach might not be surprising at a time when so many commentators write of loneliness in medical terms, referring to it as 'an epidemic'. As an example, in 2017 the former US surgeon general Vivek Murthy wrote, 'During my years caring for patients, the most common pathology I saw was not heart disease or diabetes; it was loneliness.'[18]

I absolutely know what Murthy means, but I remain uncertain about his choice of language. I have made similar observations in my own career, but I also found myself wondering whether medicine and healthcare is the most appropriate solution. This is where the debate gets tricky. There is no doubt that social issues like loneliness have a profound impact on health, but to consider healthcare without dealing with the underlying issues is to provide a second-rate service.

I can still picture one of my patients – I'll call her Brenda – who came to see me with persistent severe headaches. After many consultations and some investigations, it became clear that the cause of the problem was her dreadful relationship with her husband. She eventually left him and her headaches stopped. Were they a medical problem, or a social one?

It was understandable for her to consult a doctor, and I would have felt deficient had I not explored her psychological and social situation, as well as her physical symptoms. Trainee doctors are encouraged to explore problems in physical, psychological and social terms. But if everything impacts on health, where are the boundaries to healthcare?

I tried to address this problem in a lecture I gave back in 2006.[19] As I said at the time, 'Some of the problems that are brought to us arrive simply because we are there. They get brought to a doctor because there is almost no one else freely available to turn to.' I still find this puzzling. We have designed a model of healthcare that is all-encompassing, only to struggle with the fact. As the saying goes, 'Be careful what you wish for.'

Back in Chapter 7, I referred to those doctors who are increasingly concerned about the inappropriate medicalization of life, meaning that concepts like 'social prescribing' are coming to the fore. Social prescribing involves health professionals referring people to a range of local, non-clinical services, typically provided by voluntary and community sector organizations, and which involve activities such as volunteering, arts activities, group learning, gardening, befriending, cookery, healthy eating and a range of sports. Such social prescribing has been shown to be particularly appropriate for people with both mild or long-term mental health problems, people with complex needs, those who are socially isolated and people with multiple long-term conditions who frequently attend either primary or secondary healthcare.[20]

When Professor Dame Helen Stokes-Lampard, a former chair of the Royal College of General Practitioners in the UK, took up a new post leading a National Academy for Social Prescribing, she said in an interview that rising numbers of people were turning to their doctors for help, when their main problem was loneliness.[21] As she said, 'While our social media world has mushroomed, the people with whom we have meaningful relationships has shrunk. We used to have stronger communities.'

Stokes-Lampard described this new national initiative – which aims to involve one million patients every year by 2024 – as an attempt to rebuild connections within society. She said, 'I would argue that a form of social prescribing has always existed. It's what GPs, priests, hairdressers, bartenders, postmen and women have always done – which is recognizing someone is missing something in their life'.

There is no denying this, and the academy is a logical way forward that may have significant economic benefits. Where people have support through social prescribing, on average their GP consultations reduce by 28 per cent and their A&E attendances reduce by 24 per cent.[22]

But perhaps we need to ask *why* we are in a society where people need to access social support through the healthcare system? Is the ever-expanding role of doctors yet another side effect of the expansion of healthcare, an unintended consequence of our 'whole-person approach' to care? But if this activity *isn't* healthcare, what is it? This argument is critical to the future of care. In an ideal future, these services and this support will be readily available to citizens directly, without people necessarily feeling a need to consult a doctor or nurse. If medical practices are to function for the maximum benefit of their practice populations, these non-medical approaches will need to be core to their work. The all-too-common expectation that every problem can be treated medically and needs to be seen by a doctor or nurse must fade away. I've known friends who have been referred for these non-medical approaches and who then complain that they were 'fobbed off' – that their problem was not being treated seriously. Perhaps this attitude is an understandable legacy of a period of practice when medical treatments were always seen as the preferred way forward for almost every problem presented to a doctor. That time has surely come to an end.

In 2018, the UK government appointed a 'minister for loneliness'. Writing in the *New Yorker*, Rebecca Mead compared the idea of a plan to solve loneliness to Brexit; both, she said, were 'based on fantasy: in the case of Brexit, that a lost sovereignty can be regained without social cost; in the case of the Loneliness Ministry, that a rupture in the social fabric can be repaired on the cheap'.[23]

As Sophie McBain wrote in the *New Statesman*, the government's approach illustrates the increasing use of medicine as something that can address a spiritual, economic and political malaise. As she said, 'We may not yet be ready to think of loneliness as an illness per se, but we're starting to treat it as one, as an ailment requiring a prescription, as something pathological, as a costly public health issue.'[24]

Although loneliness is not restricted to the elderly, it is something that large numbers of elderly people experience. General practitioners in the UK report that they each see as many as five patients every day fundamentally because they are lonely. How we choose to address this issue will tell us a great deal about how we want society to function. Would we prefer to use medication or social engagement to deal with the symptoms of loneliness?

The mind and the body

Understanding the connections between social, emotional and physical health is becoming increasingly important. At present, too many elderly people experience a vicious cycle of misery. Because they are ill, they are less able to socialize with others; as a result they become increasingly isolated, which further exacerbates their illness.

A fascinating article in *Nature Reviews Neuroscience* explained the biological basis of what happens.[25] Cytokines, a form of chemical messenger in the immune system, are linked to inflammation but also change our behaviour, leading us to withdraw from social contact. From an evolutionary perspective, this makes sense.

We all know what it's like to feel unwell, particularly with an infection. As well as feeling feverish and nauseated, our behaviour changes. We are likely to ignore food and drink, to lose interest in our physical and social environments, and to feel tired, irritated and depressed, with difficulty concentrating. All these sensations are generally viewed as uncomfortable but harmless components of infections.

We are so used to these sensations that most of us don't wonder how or why they occur. In just the same way that fear is normal in the presence of an aggressive predator and makes us seek safety, so are these sensations of unwellness a normal response to infection. From an evolutionary perspective, they would have made us seek support from other people, making us much less vulnerable.

But in longer-term illnesses, this biological response may be less appropriate and helpful, especially in those people who are more emotionally or practically isolated. Over the past few years, it has been established that these cytokines induce not only symptoms of sickness, but also major depressive disorders in physically ill patients with no previous history of mental disorders. In addition, because of the lack of support, people who are more isolated tend to have more inflammation, which in turn leads to depression and stress, which leads them to withdraw further – a classic vicious cycle.

This provides more evidence that the traditional separation of the physical and the emotional aspects of our lives is a deeply flawed construct, and a recognition that social relationships can be hugely important to our physical and emotional health. And is this more than theory? A 2010 paper in *PLOS Medicine* showed that people with strong social relationships had a 50 per cent lower chance of death across the average study period than those with weak connections.[26]

Looking at this positively, we might conclude that older patients with multiple health conditions will not inevitably be more likely to die prematurely if they have strong social support. Social contact really matters, and a lack of it may well have been a major factor in the continuing escalation of healthcare costs.

The way we live can clearly have a profound effect on our health. As they become older, many people begin to question their priorities.

Age often brings multiple health problems and a multiplicity of different appointments and tests, which can become immensely time-consuming. If you add to these preventative check-ups and medications, you end up with a healthcare system that is designed to add more years to our life, but sometimes ends up taking away the life from the years. In her book *Natural Causes: Life, Death and the Illusion of Control*, the American writer Barbara Ehrenreich described how, in her mid-seventies, she gradually gave up on many medical measures, such as cancer screenings, annual check-ups and cervical smears.[27] As she wrote, 'Most of my educated middle-class friends had begun to double down on the health-related efforts at the onset of middle age, if not earlier. They undertook exercise or yoga regimens: they filled their calendars with upcoming medical tests and exams.'

Instead Ehrenreich came to realize that she was 'old enough to die'. If she was acutely ill, she would get it sorted, but she wouldn't agonise about each and every risk factor and how to avoid it. She made choices around diet and activity because she enjoyed them, not because she wanted to do things that would extend her life.

Each of us will react to this idea differently, but I think Ehrenreich makes a valid point. After all, old age is very much a phase of life rather than a disease. It isn't there to be defeated or endured. It is there for living – not just for merely existing. As we get older, the medicalization of our every waking activity feels like a curious priority. However hard we try, we can't beat the Grim Reaper; scrambling for new things that might prolong our life is no way to live. There's much more to life – and to ageing – than that.

CHAPTER 10

And in the End …

It may well be apocryphal, but there's a great story of a poster being displayed in a maternity unit to remind staff that 'The first two days of life are the most hazardous.' Someone had written on it, 'And the last two aren't too good, either.'

Birth and death are the only two certainties in every life, and yet contemporary Western culture has a tendency to forget that the second of these things is an inevitability that needs to be planned for. Dying should not be seen as failure, as what happens when medical care and treatment fails. When we are determining the needs of any healthcare system, end-of-life care should be treated as an important priority rather than being dismissed as an optional extra. There is nothing optional about dying, yet its arrival is sometimes treated as a surprise, as a failure. As an event that faces us all, it should be an important aspect of healthcare budgeting rather than a mere afterthought.

To understand contemporary attitudes to death, we can compare the funding of services that are offered at the start of life with those that are used at the end. As the chief executive of the UK charity Marie Curie, which provides care and support to people with terminal illness, said in a newspaper interview, 'Just imagine if the quality of your local maternity services depended on how much money had been raised by cake sales and sponsorship of marathon runners. We would regard this as an entirely intolerable state of affairs.' Then why, he asked, do we accept this funding model for the care that we receive at the end of our lives?[1]

In the UK, high-quality end-of-life care can be offered by many general practices, by palliative care specialists and by hospitals that have the time, training and staff necessary to give this area of care the priority that it needs. In addition, hospices currently support more than 200,000 patients and their families each year, as well as offering bereavement support to nearly 50,000 families. In light of the epidemic of multimorbidity that I've referred to throughout this book, hospices are also increasingly supporting people with multiple life-limiting conditions.

But hospices should not be the only place where death can be planned for. One of the aims of health policy in England is enabling patients to die in their preferred place, which for around four out of five people is believed to be their home.[2] Whatever the actual figures, personal preference really does matter. The national End of Life Care Strategy for England defines 'a good death' as being treated as an individual, being without pain and other symptoms, being in familiar surroundings and being in the company of family and friends.[3] The National Palliative and End of Life Care Partnership lists six ambitions for palliative and end-of-life care – that each person should be seen as an individual, that they should have fair access to care, that comfort and wellbeing are maximized, care is coordinated, all staff are prepared to care and each community is prepared to help. This really should not be too much to ask.[4]

However, recent data show that almost half of all deaths in England occur in hospital, nearly a quarter occur in people's own home, 22 per cent occur in care homes and 6 per cent occur in a hospice.[5] The majority of people want to end their lives in familiar surroundings, but many of us are denied this opportunity because of a lack of support for families, a lack of forward planning and staffing shortages.

End-of-life care should surely be a major aspect of any 'cradle-to-grave' healthcare system, but most of the funding for hospices does not come from the National Health Service. English hospices receive an average 32 per cent of their income from the government. In Scotland the figure is 38 per cent, in Northern Ireland it is 34 per cent and in Wales it is 26 per cent.[6] You might think the state would be more supportive of children's hospices, but in the UK, on average, the funding they receive from the government represents just 17 per cent of their expenditure. The rest of their funding comes from their local communities, which means charity shops, fundraising activities, legacies, hospice lotteries and investments. There's nothing wrong with the voluntary sector playing a role in any aspect of care, but I'm concerned that the state appears to regard end-of-life care as being so much less important.

Does the lack of public pressure to improve funding reflect our reluctance to think about death, even though we know it will happen to us and to our loved ones? Dying with comfort should be a basic human right, not one that depends on charity shops and the generosity of volunteers. It is also another aspect of care where inequalities are demonstrably important; the poorest patients who are terminally ill with cancer are more likely to die in hospital than the most affluent. Hospitals can be wonderful places, but they are not always equipped or designed to deal well with death, and staff do not always have the time and energy to support the needs of the dying while caring for the living. And while it is vitally important that healthcare provides the best possible quality of care when and if it is needed, there is no doubt that the natural process of dying has been overmedicalized. Healthcare can be great at treating pain or breathlessness, but it surely cannot be the best way of tackling fear or loneliness.

In the US, palliative care is one of the most rapidly growing fields of healthcare. Its benefits have been shown in multiple clinical trials: increased patient and provider satisfaction, equal or better symptom control, more discernment and honouring of a chosen place of death, fewer and less intensive hospital admissions in the last month of life, less anxiety and depression, less caregiver distress, and cost savings.[7]

The most recent statistics regarding place of death in the US show that the percentage of deaths that occurred in a hospital decreased from approximately half (50.2 per cent) in 2000 to 37.3 per cent in 2014 – a significant reduction.[8] In this time, the percentage of deaths that occurred at a decedent's home increased by nearly 30 per cent, while the percentage that occurred in hospices and all other places increased by 242.9 per cent, from 3.5 per cent to 12.0 per cent. These are quite dramatic changes.

In his wonderful book *Being Mortal*, Atul Gawande calls for a change in the way that medical professionals treat patients who are approaching the end of their life.[9] He recommends that instead of focusing on survival, practitioners should concentrate on improving quality of life and enabling wellbeing. He recognizes the negativity with which some doctors regard palliative care – after all, telling a patient that you would like them to consider being looked after in a hospice can sometimes be perceived as 'giving up' on their care. However, the fact that curative medicine may have nothing more to offer someone may be less important than the simple fact that with refocused objectives, a great deal can be done to help them. Gawande describes this as 'care with different goals' – a beautiful phrase.

Intriguingly, research shows that palliative care can actually extend some patients' lives. The reasons are uncertain, but it may be because it can help them decide to stop treatments such as chemotherapy, which can cause more harm than good towards the end of life.

There's more to treatment than cure
Many people's perceptions of medicine often fail to take into account the importance of end-of-life care. When Barbara Bush, the former first lady of the United States, was dying, media outlets reported that she had 'halted medical treatment'. The headlines were similar when the veteran US senator John McCain was dying of an aggressive brain cancer; a report from Reuters stated that he had 'chosen to discontinue medical treatment'.

However, such statements present a fundamentally misleading view of end-of-life care. Medical treatment and care at this stage in life should aim not just to cure but to support and comfort, to ease symptoms and provide dignity. Failing to cure does not mean failed treatment – it is treatment with a different, but vitally important, goal. All too often, clinicians risk putting their entire focus onto curing rather than caring. Both aspects of medical care are vital, and knowing when 'enough is enough' is an important clinical skill. As Dr Richard Smith, a former editor of the *British Medical Journal*, has noted, 'Doctors rarely want to give up.' As long as there is any possibility of diagnosis and cure, they tend to keep at it, but when this is no longer the focus, many doctors lose the drive that previously sustained their enthusiasm. As Smith says, 'As the long siege drags on, and one after another treatment has begun to fail, those enthusiasms tend to fall by the wayside. Emotionally doctors then tend to disappear; physically too, they sometimes all but disappear.'[10]

It's not just doctors who can be overly focused on cures when this is no longer appropriate – society seems to have the same problem. Writing in the *British Medical Journal,* the senior physician Dr David Oliver wrote, 'during my career, society has become ever more high-tech and "can-do" and … less willing to accept the very real limits of medicine'.[11]

Unrealistic expectations among patients and their loved ones are something that almost every doctor experiences. Indeed, the obligation to aggressively pursue a cure at a point when palliation is much kinder and more appropriate is a real downside of some contemporary medical practice. Oliver continued:

> I'm not the only doctor who has had meetings with families asking why a ninety-year-old relative who had complex multiple problems and was admitted with, say, a hip fracture, pneumonia, acute kidney injury and delirium has died. I'm also not the only one who's had discussions with families who rewrite history by claiming that patients were 'perfectly alright' and 'very independent' before admission, when in reality they were admitted acutely ill, having been deteriorating for months, increasingly struggling and dependent.

A review in the *British Medical Journal* captured the nuance that is crucial in the treatment of cancer, and the important role of palliative care:

> Medical oncology aims to increase the survival rates of patients, even at metastatic stages, in addition to reducing disease-related and treatment-related

symptoms. However, providing palliative care, which includes symptom management, nutritional support, psychosocial support and assistance with end-of-life preferences to improve quality of life, may be as important as survival issues at metastatic stages.[12]

Gawande has written, 'The lesson seems almost zen: you live longer only when you stop trying to live longer.' But what is clearly unacceptable in modern healthcare is a model of care that treats death as failure and does everything in its power to 'win'. There is nothing wrong with trying to cure cancer or other potentially life-threatening diseases, but a mindset that doesn't understand when it is good practice to focus on the quality rather than just the quantity of life is profoundly misplaced. And such decisions, of course, do not only lie with the doctor.

In the US, a national 'Coping with Cancer' project in 2008 showed that terminally ill cancer patients who were either put on a mechanical ventilator, received defibrillation or chest compressions, or were admitted to intensive care units shortly prior to their death had a significantly worse quality of life in their final week than patients who did not receive these interventions.[13] Furthermore, it's not just the patients who suffer. Six months after the death of a patient, their caregivers were three times as likely to suffer from major depression than the loved ones of patients who hadn't undergone these treatments. It depresses me to hear of very sick and elderly people being rushed to hospital from a care home to have all manner of drugs and aggressive therapies when their condition deteriorates; after all, they would probably have much preferred to stay in the place that has become their home and be treated with gentleness, kindness and symptom control. This decision should lie with the patient or their family, but all too often it is taken away from them.

The recent case of a nurse being disciplined because she had failed to carry out cardiac resuscitation on an eighty-nine-year-old terminally ill woman seems to exemplify many aspects of the problem. Great age should not automatically be treated as a terminal disease, but humanity, sensitivity, common sense and kindness are all immensely important aspects of care. As the chief executive of the UK's Nursing and Midwifery Council wrote about this particular case, it 'highlights the responsibilities of those in charge of running health and care services to ensure difficult conversations about end-of-life care take place at the appropriate time, and are clearly understood'.[14]

As the saying – attributed to Hippocrates – goes, 'Cure sometimes, treat often, comfort always.' For clinicians to treat the terminally ill with aggressive therapies simply to avoid complaint and the risk of litigation is a retrograde step. In previous generations, doctors tended to be far more willing to recognize that death was near, and far less arrogant about the chance of cure.

No one lives forever, and as we become older and frailer, the approach to treatment requires modification. A study of over 200,000 people above the age of seventy-five in England[15] showed that those who were severely frail were four times more likely to be admitted to hospital, five times more likely to die and six times more likely to enter a nursing home within a twelve-month period. Despite this, nursing homes often receive complaints when residents who are deteriorating proceed to die. One third of nursing home residents admitted acutely to hospital will die during their admission, and the signs are often all too apparent. If it is clear that they are close to the end of life, why can we not support them where they live?

Fear of complaints from families often leads patients to be admitted to hospital in the last stages of their life, even when they are clearly dying. For many patients with a terminal illness, spending their final days in an intensive care unit is not what they would choose. In this scenario, the end of life arrives with little chance to say goodbye or to express the intimate, personal things we would hope to say. The priorities of terminally ill patients often include avoiding suffering, strengthening their relationships with their family and friends, not being a burden on others and remaining mentally aware – simply prolonging their life is not so important.

Sadly, our system of technological medical care often fails to meet these needs. We seem to somehow offer care that is simultaneously more expensive and less effective. Although much of this book is about the increasing cost of healthcare, I must be clear that I am *not* saying that care should be restricted *because* it is expensive – I am saying our focus should be on the needs of patients. A treatment that is expensive and highly technical will not automatically be the best option for every patient. As the distinguished doctor and writer Richard Lehman has written, 'We do not have a divine mandate to make everybody live longer. We have a human mandate to listen to people and fulfil their wishes for what remains of their lives.'[16]

Truly patient-centred

We should offer the optimum, patient-centred care simply because it is the right thing to do. If a society has limited funds – as all do – it should focus on the best ways of delivering the very best care – and instead of spending hundreds of thousands of pounds or dollars on 'me-too' drugs that combine greater cost with minimal benefit, it would surely be better to invest in greater access to high-quality palliative care.

Furthermore, as we have already seen, the benefits of highly expensive drugs can be exceedingly limited. As a 2017 *British Medical Journal* editorial stated, among the thirty-six approvals of cancer drugs made by the US Food and Drug Administration between 2008 and 2012, only five were ultimately shown to improve survival compared with existing treatments or placebo.[17] A European study confirmed these disappointing findings.[18] Of thirty-nine cancer drugs approved by the European Medicines Agency between 2009 and 2013, 57 per cent of them had no supporting evidence of better survival or improved quality of life when they went on the market. After a median 5.9 years on the market, just six of these thirty-nine agents had been shown to improve survival or quality of life.

Indeed, even when aggressive treatment *does* succeed in prolonging life, it can all too often simultaneously increase suffering. There are occasions when medicine sometimes appears to treat the body and not the person. Is that what society wants?

While I'm arguing for a different approach in order to show greater humanity rather than to save money, many cancer therapies are massively expensive. At the time of the European Cancer Medicines Agency study in 2017, it was estimated that the average cancer drug cost more than $100,000 per year of treatment – and yet their benefits can be far from certain. In the US, Medicare is legally required to pay for any drug approved by the FDA without negotiation on price, while the UK National Institute for Health and Care Excellence states that drugs that provide only marginal or uncertain benefits at high cost should not routinely be used in the NHS.

As the *BMJ* editorial stated, 'the expense and toxicity of cancer drugs means we have an obligation to expose patients to treatment only when they can reasonably expect an improvement in survival or quality of life'. We need to encourage innovation, of course, but not at absurd levels of cost.

Meanwhile, palliative care continues to be financed by bake sales, charity coffee mornings and sponsored runs – the contrast could not be greater. A colossal £500 million is spent each year on cancer research, while a derisory £5.49 million goes towards researching end-of-life care. We need research into cancer treatments, of course – science must advance – but not at the cost of delivering care to those who need it. It's not as if we have made a conscious decision to spend a fortune on a number of barely effective drugs that are offered, sometimes inappropriately, at the end of life, while failing to deliver the investment in community and primary care that keeps being promised, but never appears. Is this really how our society would like its funds to be prioritized?

As Sarah Scobie, the deputy director of research at the Nuffield Trust, has said: 'If this trend is set to stay and more people are choosing to die or be cared for at home, then it represents a significant shift in demand for healthcare, and more focus will be needed to ensure families, patients and carers at home have the right support.'[19] Our changing demography means that the situation is only going to get worse. Today there are 1.6 million people aged over eighty-five, but this is expected to double over the next twenty-five years. This wonderful achievement for humankind will mean that many more of us will have multiple health problems in our final days, and it is clear that our current healthcare systems are not geared up to cope. We should ignore the problem at our peril.

CHAPTER 11

Care in the Future

The potential developments for the future of healthcare are remarkable. Consider the joint press conference held by the US president Bill Clinton and the UK prime minister Tony Blair on 26 June 2000 to mark the first sequencing of the human genome. President Clinton made his views clear, announcing that 'With this profound new knowledge, humankind is on the verge of gaining immense new power to heal. Genome science will ... revolutionize the diagnosis, prevention and treatment of most, if not all, human diseases.'[1]

That was quite a claim, but it's not an unusual one. In recent times, we have been promised innumerable exciting developments in the world of healthcare, including the following:

- Every citizen will have their full genome sequenced and analysed, so that they know their health-related risks, and how best to minimize them, almost from birth
- Treatments will be highly personalized to the individual patient
- Regular blood tests will pick up the earliest hint of cancer in advance of any symptoms, so that action can be taken pre-emptively

- Apps, smartphones and implantable devices will ensure that heart rate, blood pressure, breathing, weight and activity levels can be streamed constantly to healthcare professionals, so that feedback can optimise our health
- Our urine and faeces will be analysed automatically through smart toilets
- Robots will care for the aged and infirm

Whether you look at developments like these with enthusiasm, cynicism or horror, we can be sure both that nothing will quite work out as planned and that the cost will be almost incalculable.

As we have seen throughout this book, life-changing advances are generally followed by new problems. If our expectation is that we will live healthily and happily until the age of 150, followed by a brief illness and a painless death, then we need to become a lot more realistic. The Covid-19 pandemic has perfectly demonstrated the sorts of challenges that will always face us. Humankind has always dreamt about eliminating sickness and pain, and there's nothing wrong with dreaming – as long as we don't use it for budgetary forecasting.

While many of these ideas might have great potential, I'm confident that anyone who picks up this book in ten years' time will be astonished at how breathtakingly ignorant I turned out to be. When it comes to predicting the future, the simple fact is that no one, not even the tech gurus in Apple and Google's Silicon Valley headquarters, knows what's going to happen.

Today's speed of technological change is quite astonishing. It was just over forty years ago that Sony's portable cassette player the Walkman was regarded as the height of technological achievement, and such technology now feels impossibly dated. The first iPhone was launched as recently as 2007, and the developments since then have been extraordinary. The more we use such technologies, the more we take their existence for granted. Indeed, some of us are now inclined to complain that our human rights have been infringed if we don't get at least a 4G phone signal. An astounding new development one year can be old hat the next.

When it comes to future-scoping, we can know what is planned and what we might hope for, but it is hard to know much more than that. A quotation that has been ascribed to everyone from Samuel Goldwyn and Mark Twain to ancient Chinese scholars sums up the problem: 'You can predict anything except the future.' As the businessman Peter Drucker wrote, 'Trying to predict the future is like trying to drive down a country road at night with no lights while looking out the back window.' Our only real experience comes from looking backwards with a sense of hindsight, and we try to use this perspective to figure out what the forward view might become.

One thing we do know is how little human beings have changed. We read the plays and poems of William Shakespeare, written over 400 years ago, and recognize the universal truth in the human relationships he describes. The language may now seem outdated, but the emotions are not. Why might they change in the next hundred years? Will humans no longer worry when they become sick? Will they no longer need a human being to trust, a hand to hold? However brilliant and advanced our technology may become, our need for humanity will persist. If we get rid of that from our healthcare systems, whether on economic grounds or out of a desire for efficiency, we will lose the 'care' aspect of healthcare. And we will do that at our peril.

We can be certain about the continued need for kindness and compassion, but apart from that we have little idea what the future has in store. When I started writing this book, no one had ever heard of Covid-19. Some experts had predicted that similar viruses were likely to cause problems at some point, but we didn't know where and when. In what seemed like a matter of weeks, this coronavirus went from an interesting but distant minor concern to the greatest threat to global public health and prosperity since the Second World War. As I write these words, I have no idea what impact it will have had by the time you read them, but it is clear that the pandemic has already led to rapid and profound change in the way medicine is practised. Concepts such as online consulting that had been discussed for years but were always deemed too complex to deliver were adopted overnight. As Rahm Emanuel, chief of staff to US president Barack Obama, once said: 'You never want a serious crisis to go to waste… It's an opportunity to do things that you think you could not do before.'

However, while we will inevitably be wrong about the specifics of technological change, a number of trends are bound to have a massive impact on healthcare. We are in the middle of what might be termed the fourth industrial revolution. It is the era of cyber-physical systems, in which computers are directly integrated with physical processes – examples being as simple as cleaning robots through to medical devices such as blood glucose monitors linked to automated insulin pumps. Advances in technologies like sensors, artificial intelligence, regenerative medicine and new aspects of drug discovery have the potential to deliver a step change in the efficacy of health interventions. Each of these new developments will turn out to have significant unintended consequences, both positive and negative, and understanding what they might be is a key aspect of any attempt to plan for the future. I am not intending to undervalue new developments, but a lifetime's experience has taught me to try to be realistic – the proponents of any new advance rarely consider the potential for negative consequences.

Whenever I've discussed new policy proposals with British health ministers, I've suggested that they give a small group of advisers a week to consider just how the proposals might go wrong because, as sure as eggs is eggs, that is what will happen in the real world. However, people rarely listen – they are too bound up in the excitement of potential benefits to consider potential risks.

A relatively simple example from the recent past has been the introduction of electronic medical record systems. From the inception of NHS general practice in the UK, medical records were always written on pieces of card that were stored in what were called 'Lloyd George envelopes'. As medicine became more complex and searching for information became more challenging, the solution lay in computerized medical records.

This solved many record-related problems. Instead of thumbing through cards in search of a blood pressure result, for example, a couple of taps on the computer keyboard would yield the answer. Charts and trends could be plotted, and the result was much greater efficiency. If research showed problems with a drug, every doctor with a patient who might be taking it could identify and notify them with a couple of clicks. The systems were efficient and easy to use, with minimal downsides. A real win for technology.

In 2004, the UK government solved a crisis in the recruitment of British GPs through the offer of a very significant pay rise, but ministers felt – entirely reasonably – that family doctors should have to justify this extra income. New payments were to be made against outcomes and activity that would be measured through the Quality and Outcomes Framework (QOF), with GPs presenting data to demonstrate that their care was of an appropriate quality.

In this contract, a GP practice could accumulate 'QOF points' depending on their level of achievement in 146 indicators, such as the proportion of patients with coronary heart disease whose cholesterol was measured, or the number of patients with depression who had answered a standard questionnaire on severity. At the end of the financial year, the number of points achieved by the practice was converted into a payment.

Here we have two straightforward initiatives – computerized records and a quality-based contract – both introduced for entirely logical, worthwhile and positive reasons. What could possibly go wrong? Well, ask almost any patient describing almost any consultation with almost any doctor in the UK in the last few years. All too often they might say, 'He spent more time looking at the computer screen than looking at me,' or, 'She was more interested in making sure I'd had my blood pressure recorded than finding out what I was worried about.'

I'll never forget a patient of mine, a man in his early fifties with high blood pressure, who came to see me for a routine review. To my shame, I can recall that as I scrolled through his records on the computer with my back to him, I suddenly became aware that he was crying. As soon as I realized, I turned to him, apologized and turned my computer off. The technology and the prioritization of the bio-medical over the human had got in the way of what mattered in that consultation. It was another classic side effect, and it taught me an important lesson: research is clear that patient satisfaction is closely linked to a sense of being listened to; anything that might interfere with that can have serious negative effects.

None of this is any reason to abandon new technology – we don't have to choose between the technical and the human. Indeed, we absolutely need both – and this means being alert for unintended consequences, rather than pretending that they don't exist in our rush for progress. An understanding of both the ergonomics and the human factors involved in healthcare consultations is critical – we mustn't assume that a new way of working will only bring benefits.

If we assume that the future will be nothing like we expect, what are the new developments that are likely to have a major impact on healthcare delivery and cost? The key ones might be artificial intelligence, robotics, genomics and personalized medicines, and the first two of these could be summed up by the term 'new technologies'.

New technologies

Humankind has long been anxious about machines undertaking tasks that might previously have been carried out by humans. Today, artificial intelligence and robotics are pushing the boundaries of what can be automated, not just in relation to manual work but also in more complex cognitive tasks. A US report from 2013 found that almost half of occupations have aspects of the job that are vulnerable to automation, including many areas of healthcare.[2] While it is clear that genuine creativity, thinking on your feet and interpreting social cues is hard to automate, many healthcare roles, such as the screening of large numbers of X-rays or pathology samples, would seem well suited to automation. However, final diagnostic decisions are likely to require humans for some time yet.

The global healthcare expert Mark Britnell has shown that by 2030, there will be a worldwide need for 80 million people working in healthcare, while the World Health Organization has estimated that there will be a shortage of around 18 million workers.[3] Britnell believes that this shortfall might be made up in a number of ways, including sensitively harnessing the power of robotics. It is clear that simply recruiting staff from other countries that need clinical staff themselves is no longer the solution.

In many scenarios, automation in healthcare will clearly be focused on supporting professionals rather than replacing them. The challenge will then be in how to rethink the work that people do, redesigning roles to make them more sustainable and meaningful – in other words, the things that humans are best at. Indeed, more technology should mean that we can achieve *more* complex and creative decision-making on the healthcare frontline, the opposite of what might be feared. A technological approach, far from condemning us to being seen as the implementers of algorithms, could and should permit the reverse.

As an example, receptionists in primary care could become less focused on clerical work and instead be freed up to focus more on patient interaction. The supporting role of automation is particularly important if it can be used to address workloads that are becoming increasingly unmanageable. A study in 2019 showed that around 44 per cent of administrative tasks in general practice could be automated, though the report stressed that what might seem to be a simple clerical task may be much more complex on a human level. As it stated:

> Some tasks with high automatability scores will be challenging to implement for social and organizational reasons. Previous research has shown that staff contribute to patient quality and safety through hidden ways that emerge in the moment and require tacit knowledge ... work, such as reading social cues, currently lies outside the capabilities of automated systems and machine learning technologies.[4]

Online consulting

For at least a decade, the potential for more healthcare to be carried out digitally was promoted by a small group of tech enthusiasts but rejected by a much larger group of sceptics who worried that practicalities, not to mention patient resistance, were almost insuperable. However, Covid-19 made online consulting the norm and face-to-face the exception – indeed, the rapidity with which healthcare has taken up digital consulting has been one potentially positive side effect of the pandemic. It has benefits on many fronts – it is time-saving for patients and clinicians, efficient, environmentally beneficial and a great aid to patient empowerment. It has also been absolutely necessary – at the height of the pandemic, it was the only way that much of the NHS could continue safely. It was also fascinating to observe how resistant some patient groups were to it, encouraged by campaigns in the news media. While some delighted in the convenience and speed that digital consulting could offer, others appeared to feel that anything other than a face-to-face appointment with a GP meant that they were being fobbed off with second-rate care. When he was UK Secretary of State for Health, Matt Hancock had been quoted as saying that all GP appointments should be done remotely by default unless a patient needed to be seen in person.[5] Subsequent media campaigns led his successor Sajid Javid to emphasize the importance of face-to-face contact and strongly criticise doctors who failed to offer it – whether appropriately or not. The future of digital consulting is far from clear.

It seems likely that in the long term, many patients will find digital consulting a valuable tool – particularly in replacing absurd outpatient reviews that effectively go: 'How are you getting on?'

'Fine thanks.' 'Excellent – I'll see you in six months.' However, much of medicine is infinitely more complex than that. I lost count of the number of consultations in my career that included a hand-on-the-door-handle 'While I'm here, doctor' request from a patient, with the real cause of their concern only being revealed after true human interaction. I'm not sure if this same sense of ease and trust will easily follow a video call; a mixture of face-to-face and virtual consultations will surely be the ideal.

While enhancing our efficiency, we must ensure that we retain aspects of care such as kindness, calmness and empathy. This doesn't mean abandoning digital and reverting to how things were in the past; we just have to ensure that 'care' is built into how we use the systems – and that certainly won't happen by accident. As Professor Martin Marshall, chair of the Royal College of General Practitioners, has written:

> If the trusting relationship between a patient and a health professional were a drug, we would marvel at its effectiveness and NICE would mandate its use in every consultation. When I'm seeing a patient who I know and who trusts me, research evidence suggests that, in comparison with a patient with whom I have no relationship, the patient will be more satisfied, more likely to engage with my advice, more likely to disclose their concerns, more likely to take up preventative and health education offers and less likely to attend the emergency department or (for older patients) be admitted to hospital. They are even, remarkably, more likely to live longer … The focus on transactions and the emphasis on efficiency is having the opposite of the

desired effect – a less effective and a less efficient health system.[6]

It is too early to know how access through digital technology will impact on our healthcare systems. If contacting a healthcare professional is as straightforward as consulting 'Dr Google', perhaps patients will make contact far more frequently. Equally possibly, if automated replies, bots and new technologies deal with a majority of initial requests, it could reduce the number of consultations. Smart apps may help improve patient engagement and enable healthcare professionals to focus on the problems that really matter. However, despite all this, we can be less certain of what the impact on affordability might be. There is also a risk of a digital divide, with certain subgroups of the population feeling less comfortable using digital methods; this may lead to a widening of health inequalities.

Big data and artificial intelligence
Modern technologies give us the opportunity to collect and analyse data on an infinitely greater scale than at any time in the past. Over the past few decades, there has been much discussion of how precision medicine might help prevent sickness and even death, resulting in early diagnosis through the identification of potential risk factors in healthy people.

The term 'big data' can be used to describe many different data-intensive technologies. Future developments will mean the ability to collect data without the need for existing methodologies such as cameras, GPS trackers and heart monitors. The next step might be smart contact lenses, implantable microchips or even 'wearable' sensors embedded in clothes. Instead of occasional medical check-ups, our health could be constantly monitored. It is too early to tell whether this will lead to a more cost-effective healthcare system. Will the benefits be outweighed by the unintended consequences? Will technology bring a healthy utopia, or an anxiety-ridden existence?

People who are enthusiastic about screening based on these technologies claim that they will enable an unprecedented monitoring of the human body. The assumption is that it will be beneficial, but there is also a considerable risk that it would increase the potential for overdiagnosis and all the harm that comes with it. As a paper in the *British Medical Journal* pointed out:

> The main problem for big data screening is that monitoring many of the features of the body with highly sensitive technologies is bound to detect many abnormalities but without the ability to tell which, if any, will become clinically manifest. As a result more people may be labelled with harmless conditions.[7]

As we have only recently started to collect data from sensors such as smartwatches, we do not yet know which abnormalities really matter. There is no doubt that with long-term research, better algorithms and machine learning, we will improve our understanding and determine what can safely be ignored. Until then, however, there is a real risk that overdiagnosis will increase anxiety levels, which in itself can be detrimental to health. As ever, the issues are not straightforward.

Even if the collection of personal data is shown to increase the accuracy of diagnosis, the previous bungled implementation of IT projects in the UK – such as the National Programme for IT, which cost £10 billion and was described by the government's Public Accounts Committee as 'one of the worst and most expensive contracting fiascos in public sector history' – has caused people to question whether their data might be protected. Many also wonder whether those people who make decisions might be putting private profit before the public interest. If our data is to be used, we need much better civic engagement and a more honest debate about the benefits and risks.

But the use of big data is still in its infancy. Dan Ariely, professor of psychology and behavioural economics at Duke University, compared it to teenage sex – 'everyone talks about it, nobody really knows how to do it, everyone thinks everyone else is doing it, so everyone claims they are doing it'.[8]

Like big data, artificial intelligence is seen as having great potential in medicine and healthcare. Rather than replacing doctors and other clinicians, it should allow them to spend more time doing the tasks that only humans can do, a genuine benefit. Indeed, many tasks that are currently done by clinicians could be eased dramatically by the use of AI – particularly the initial reading of scans and some aspects of laboratory work.

Medical specialties that rely on imaging data have already begun to show benefits from the implementation of AI methods.[9] Within radiology, AI appears to be particularly effective at recognizing complex patterns in imaging data and can provide a quantitative assessment in an automated fashion. However, this works best when it is used as a tool that assists doctors rather than replacing them entirely.

All this is likely to have beneficial impacts on cost, though this is not guaranteed. If tests become cheaper and easier to use, will they be used more frequently? And if they are, will this be entirely beneficial or a further source of overdiagnosis and overtreatment? The key lies in constant research and review, but the hope must be that in the long run, AI can bring together the advantages of people and computers.

Robotics

Robotics will impact healthcare in numerous ways. The most significant are surgical robots (particularly focusing on minimally invasive procedures), exoskeletons (designed to assist the rehabilitation of patients with lower limb disorders, including those caused by spinal cord injuries and strokes), care robots (designed to provide care and support to elderly and disabled patients), and hospital robots, which are used to deliver medications, laboratory specimens or other sensitive material within a hospital, and even to disinfect hospital devices and equipment.

The idea of using technology to support human professionals is nothing new. Nevertheless, many attempts to replace people with machines in manufacturing industries turned out to be less successful than was originally hoped; even though robots have superhuman strength and don't tire, they currently lack the dexterity, agility and flexibility of humans.[10] This ultimately gave rise to the concept of collaborative robots, or 'cobots', that paired human skills with robotic benefits.

This idea that new technology could support rather than replace humans must be the most positive way of using it. After all, humanity is fundamental to healthcare. However technically adept they might be, computers are highly unlikely to be able to care for and communicate with patients, skills that require a high degree of social and emotional intelligence. We are a very long way from developing computers that have such abilities.

That said, robots have been shown to be a useful support in the care of the elderly. In an international trial, they were able to hold simple conversations, which boosted patients' mental health and reduced loneliness. The wheeled robots, which move independently and gesture with robotic arms, are designed to be 'culturally competent', which means that they can be programmed to learn about the interests of care home residents. However, while they may be able to initiate rudimentary conversations, play residents' favourite music and offer practical help including medicine reminders,[11] they should certainly not ever replace human beings. When I'm dying, I don't want to have my hand held by a robot – it would be as empathic as the computer-generated apology of a late-running train or a greeting we might hear from Alexa or Siri. In addition, the importance of human touch is easy to underestimate. The early phases of the Covid pandemic, with the focus on social distancing, made this all too clear – particularly to those in hospitals or care homes who were denied even the touch of family members. Research has demonstrated that touch enhances feelings of safety and trust; basic warm touch calms cardiovascular stress by activating the vagus nerve, which is intimately involved with our compassionate response. Indeed, a simple touch can trigger the release of oxytocin, a hormone that acts as a chemical messenger and has an important role in many human behaviours including sexual arousal, recognition, trust, romantic attachment and mother–infant bonding.[12] It seems unlikely that the touch of a robot could ever provide the same benefits.

There is also the risk that as robotic technology becomes more sophisticated, the work of healthcare assistants may become easier to automate. Jobs like monitoring patients' vital signs and serving meals might sound ideally placed for robotics. However, performing this type of task enables healthcare assistants to pick up on patients' problems and to provide necessary emotional human support; we're taking a risk if we underestimate the importance of such contact.

As for the impact of all this on healthcare costs, direct costs are likely to fall if technology replaces humans but satisfaction may fall too, meaning poorer outcomes or increased consultation. Robotics is a technology that is likely to be cost-effective, but its unintended consequences are currently massively unclear.

Genomics and molecular biology
The 2017 annual report of the chief medical officer for England was titled 'Generation Genome'.[13] In its introduction, Professor Dame Sally Davies wrote:

> Genomics is not tomorrow. It's here today. I believe genomic services should be available to more patients, while being a cost-effective service in the NHS. This is exciting science with the potential for fantastic improvements in prevention, health protection and patient outcomes. Now we need to welcome the genomic era and deliver the genomic dream!

There is no doubt that the ability to analyse someone's genetic constitution at the level of the entire genome (meaning 3.2 billion 'letters' of DNA's molecular code) will significantly transform some aspects of healthcare. An astonishing achievement, it will improve cancer care and help to identify rare and debilitating genetic diseases, and it should lead to new medicines and treatments. Unlike so many other medical technologies, the cost of carrying out full genome analysis has dropped dramatically. The estimated cost for generating the initial 'draft' human genome sequence was about $300 million. Since then, the price of genetic sequencing has fallen at an astonishing speed, from $50,000 a decade ago to roughly $600 today. The Chinese firm BGI recently claimed to have created a system that can sequence a full genome for just $100. It is clear that the challenge is going to shift from the affordability of sequencing to knowing how to use its answers.

One distinct benefit will lie in improved diagnosis, particularly for the 6 per cent of the population who have rare inherited diseases and who often struggle to get a clear diagnosis. A preliminary report on the UK's 100,000 Genomes Project, published in the *New England Journal of Medicine*, analysed the diagnostic and clinical impact of genetic sequencing within a national healthcare system.[14] The researchers analysed the genomes of nearly 5,000 people from over 2,000 families looking for rare genetic variants that might explain their conditions, and this led to a new diagnosis in a quarter of patients. This in itself can be beneficial – it is usually helpful to know what condition you might have – and a quarter of these people subsequently received more focused care. Indeed, for a number of conditions, including intellectual disability, vision and hearing disorders, the diagnostic yield was even higher, at between 40 and 55 per cent.

While we are in the earliest days of this technology, the benefits of knowing which individuals are at the highest risk of developing particular conditions, such as coronary heart disease or stroke, are clear. We currently have to treat large numbers of patients in the knowledge that some of them will benefit; in the future, we may be able to identify *which* individuals are the most likely to benefit from treatment, saving many others from having to take medication unnecessarily. The question of how this will affect the pharmaceutical industry's business model then arises. If medication is currently given to fifty people in order to benefit one of them, what would the drug need to cost if it was given to a far smaller number of patients? And how would that affect its profitability?

The issue of using genomics to predict risk raises questions about privacy and the ownership and commercialization of an individual's genetic data, not to mention the ethical difficulties that may result. Not everyone will want to know if their genetic make-up suggests that they are at risk of developing a particular condition, and genetic counsellors may well struggle to explain these complex issues. Politicians have enthused about the potential benefits of the current GRAIL study – a multi-cancer early detection test that aims to detect over fifty types of cancers with a single blood test. While this may have great potential, it is vital that research fully covers the ethical and practical issues, as well as the purely scientific ones.[15]

Many doctors are struggling to advise patients about the genetic testing that is already carried out by private companies. A paper in the *British Medical Journal* pointed out that finding a 'health risk' via direct-to-consumer genetic testing often does not mean that a patient will go on to develop the health problem in question – such genetic tests can report false positives, while 'reassuring' results might be false negatives.[16] This can be an emotional, practical and ethical nightmare.

Nevertheless, even a UK health secretary, Matt Hancock, demonstrated an intriguing mix of ignorance and over-enthusiasm when talking about the potential of genetic testing. Ahead of a speech at the Royal Society, Hancock discussed his decision to establish his risk of developing a number of medical conditions through a commercial genetic test. The results had indicated that his chance of developing prostate cancer before he was seventy-five was apparently almost 15 per cent, and he was quoted as saying that he planned to arrange further screening. However, this comment was met with derision from many clinicians and statisticians – as one geneticist observed, 'There is no such thing as a screening appointment for prostate cancer. We don't do them because they don't work; they're a waste of time and money.'

Other experts pointed out that although Hancock had described his 15 per cent lifetime risk of prostate cancer as 'high', it was only marginally above the population average risk of 12 per cent. Analysing risk through genomics is only part of the challenge – communicating it is much harder. How an individual responds to being told their risk for a condition is high – or even low – may have a profound impact on how they live their life. Genomics Plc, the Oxford-based company that provided Hancock with his risk scores, states on its website that 'We can identify individuals at risk of particular diseases, and pinpoint subsets of patients who will benefit from tailored interventions via therapeutics or lifestyle changes.'

Knowing your personal risk may also have a significant impact on your ability to obtain healthcare insurance. The fact that this will always be kept confidential counts for nothing if the application process requires an individual to declare everything they know about themselves. As a report from the Swiss Re Institute stated:

> Insurers are aware that there are some risks with the increased availability of genetic information. Most prominent of these is an information asymmetry. If individuals have access to genetic data that their insurer does not, it could be the basis of non-disclosure and anti-selection.[17]

For those who see an insurance model as being the solution to healthcare funding, the impact of genomics and genetic testing needs to be very clearly addressed. Genomics is still in its infancy, but there is no doubt that it has extraordinary potential. The verdict is still out on how it might impact on healthcare provision and costs. It may, in time, allow for better-targeted screening, and it is likely to have a particularly important impact on the care of patients with cancer.

Cancer is a complex condition. Even the cancer that affects one particular organ is actually a multiplicity of different conditions, each of which may respond differently to treatment. Understanding more about the genetic profile of a cancer patient may well help to unravel which treatments are most likely to be successful. Indeed, some potentially effective drugs only work on a small subset of the population and cause severe side effects in others. If we can identify that subset in advance, it will make the drugs' use more viable.

Some people believe that this increasing focus on the individual – what can be termed 'me medicine' – is developing to the detriment of 'we medicine', public health programmes such as flu immunization or childhood vaccination.[18] There is no doubt that on a global level, the public health approach has caused the biggest increase in life expectancy. Even today, countries with more social provision of healthcare and less individualistic attitudes have better health outcomes.

However, we should not have to choose between individual treatment and public health. Healthcare systems need to address issues at the macro level while also receiving the potential benefits of personalized approaches to cancer treatment that are making the illness more survivable. New research tools such as rapid gene sequencing have allowed the development of much more specific cancer treatment, a trend that will no doubt continue.

In the last ten years, a whole new branch of cancer therapy has been developed that harnesses the immune system's response to the illness. Chimeric antigen receptor T-cell therapy is a new treatment that involves the T-cells – cells that fight off bacteria and virus infections – being reprogrammed to identify certain cancer cells directly. In other words, the body's immune system is harnessed to attack the cancer. It is a highly complex and potentially risky treatment, but it has been shown to be effective in trials, including where other available treatments have failed.

Our biggest challenge lies in working out how to pay for such therapy. It might have the potential to be extraordinarily effective, but it is also hugely expensive. In 2019, the list price in the UK for tisagenlecleucel was £282,000. In the US, a 2019 report stated that hospitals might need to charge as much as $1.5 million for it, to avoid losing money.[19]

While there has been an unprecedented wave of investment and innovation, the question of whether the average healthcare system will be able to provide such drugs for anyone who needs them remains. The use of clearly defined criteria to determine how these remarkable drugs can best be used will be critical. Otherwise, only the richest – or those with the most influence – will benefit.

CHAPTER 12

A Way Forward

The problems are clear, but is there a solution?

With demand for care increasing, costs escalating, populations growing and expectations rising, and all while economies are facing a desperate struggle to source sufficient funding, what possible solutions might there be? After all, there do *have* to be solutions. If this challenge isn't tackled, we will end up either with increasing waiting times, reductions in the quality of care or with the most expensive care being restricted to those who are able to pay – not a recipe for a cohesive, happy and functioning society.

There is no doubt that the Covid-19 pandemic has had – and will continue to have – a profound impact on healthcare systems around the world. Health has taken precedence over every other aspect of life, but pandemics are not the norm. They are short-term emergencies, and while plans can be put in place to deal with them, no system could tolerate the massive levels of spending that might be required in the long term. In addition, the pandemic has highlighted the challenges that result when demand exceeds resources. Finding solutions became a matter of life and death.

In the early days of the pandemic in northern Italy, doctors were called on to make unimaginably tough decisions as to which patients could be treated when there were simply not enough beds and respirators to go around. A doctor working in one of Milan's largest hospitals said, 'It is a fact that we will have to choose [whom to treat], and this choice will be entrusted to individual operators on the ground who may find themselves facing ethical problems.'[1] This was no theoretical exercise, and it shone a light on the challenges we have seen throughout this book.

However, this global catastrophe may also provide a natural pivot point – an opportunity to rethink, and maybe to start anew. We simply cannot carry on as we were before – and while some people think the long-term answer is to continue the massive healthcare spending that was needed in the early days of the pandemic, this is simply unsustainable and ignores the urgent requirements of other aspects of public life.

So what is the solution? In democracies, the budgetary approach of governments tends to be based on what is most likely to be acceptable to the electorate. In Chapter 2, I described how difficult it is to deliver quality, affordability and access simultaneously, at least without significant changes to the way services are delivered. This is not just an issue for politicians – it is an issue for the whole of society, whether we are patients, clinicians, academics, industrialists or citizens. It is key that any change must be based on evidence. The decision-making process should be as transparent as possible, and it must involve service users as well as clinicians and managers.

In Chapter 1, I used the analogy of diagnosing and treating anaemia to demonstrate how society might address inadequate healthcare funding. In treating the condition, you should only prescribe iron if deficiency of it is actually the problem. If there is a different cause, extra iron may end up being completely wasted, and it might even be harmful. It is the same with healthcare funding. While more money is always useful – and will be essential in addressing the waiting lists that built up during the pandemic, exacerbated by the previous impact of austerity – it is not necessarily the only solution.

Some of the challenges this book has described include a lack of clarity as to the ultimate aspirations of care, an excessive focus on single conditions at a time when many of us have multiple long-term conditions, and the outdated hospital-led paradigm for healthcare. We've looked at waste, overtreatment and overdiagnosis, increasing expectations of healthcare and the puzzling situation whereby populations that have never been healthier are nevertheless increasingly concerned about health issues. We've noted that medical solutions may be used for non-medical issues, the ever-increasing costs of pharmaceuticals, underinvestment in public health measures and the challenge posed when very expensive therapies for small numbers of patients are prioritized over comfort and care for much larger numbers of patients. That's quite a list.

Solutions

No single solution will address all these issues, but a great deal could be done to address some of them. This might begin with an acceptance that for all its successes, healthcare has lost its way and needs to refocus. It will also require a greater clarity around the ultimate aim of medical care. Throughout history, there has been a constant and futile fight with mortality. Just as every generation looks back with astonishment at the weapons that its predecessors chose to use in this fight, future generations will look at us in just the same way.

And the information age will have a profound effect on healthcare, as it has on everything else. For centuries, the medical profession held all the knowledge, just as priests had held all the power prior to the Reformation. Explaining the meaning of the Bible, which was written in Latin, to ordinary people was an essential part of the role of the priesthood.[2] The clergy made it clear that years of training were needed to understand the text, and that it would be dangerous to let the general public loose on such material. When the scriptures were eventually translated into English, the relationship between clergy and laity changed dramatically.

The impact of the internet on the medical world has been just as significant. While society will always require doctors to help citizens understand and interpret the complexities of the science, as well as to deliver care when needed, medicine should be done *with* people rather than *to* them. And now that all the knowledge in the world is available to anyone with access to a computer or smartphone, the clinical professions will never again be its only source – but they will still need to be trusted, trustworthy and caring in its interpretation and application.

Furthermore, for the last few generations, healthcare has been led by hospitals. In most Western countries, prestige in the medical profession has become attached to specialism. Specialist expertise has become dominant, and as a result resources have flowed to hospitals to the extent that they have become the shorthand term for a political discussion of healthcare.

But the arrival of the information age, allied to the significant increase in multimorbidity, has changed everything. For the reasons I have discussed, it is no longer logical for hospitals to consume the vast majority of healthcare resources, particularly at the expense of community care and public health. We should also question the logic of spending huge sums of money on a few patients while depriving many others of care for their ongoing – but less dramatic – conditions, particularly in old age.

If healthcare systems are to flourish, there must be a far greater emphasis on self-care, and on care from family, friends and the community. A patient with diabetes spends around 0.02 per cent of their year in contact with the NHS, which probably equates to four thirty-minute consultations. That leaves 99.98 per cent of their time having to deal with the reality of living with diabetes.[3] So far, the NHS has been poor at supporting many aspects of self-care. Greater access to support through information technology will assist this partnership, as the uptake of digital consulting during the Covid-19 pandemic showed. The absurd demarcation between healthcare and social care must also be addressed. The suffering caused by Alzheimer's disease is just as challenging as the suffering caused by cancer, but at the time of writing, only one of these conditions receives healthcare funding in England. How can this be moral, ethical or kind?

As a result of these problems, the potential exists for a great deal of healthcare delivery to change in a positive and progressive way. In most countries, many long-term conditions such as type 1 diabetes are followed up through hospital outpatient visits, which cost time and money but offer minimal benefit. Conducting this traditional follow-up digitally would save both time and cut costs, as well as helping to empower patients.

Almost every commentator on the future of healthcare mentions the importance of greater engagement by patients and the public with their own health. Back in 2001, the UK Chancellor of the Exchequer Gordon Brown commissioned a long-term review of the UK National Health Service.[4] The report by Derek Wanless not only made it clear that the system needed large and sustained funding increases, but also emphasized the need for the service to engage more effectively with its users. In what the report described as a 'fully engaged scenario', levels of public engagement in relation to their health would be high. A dramatic improvement in public health, with a sharp decline in key risk factors such as smoking and obesity, would be a key element of this change.

Two years later, Wanless followed up his original report with 'Securing Good Health for the Whole Population', a review that identified the need for an increase in the availability of advice and information, established principles for public health expenditure decisions and recommended an increase in the skills and capacity of the public health workforce. If the public did not become more engaged in their care, he felt the NHS would become unsustainable. Since that time, investment in public health has shrunk.

In 2017, a King's Fund study entitled 'What Does the Public Think of the NHS?' showed that 65 per cent of the population believed that keeping healthy was primarily down to the individual, with only 7 per cent feeling that it was an NHS responsibility. The question of obligations is packed with ethical and practical difficulties. There is no doubt that if any healthcare system is to thrive, patients and the public need to take responsibility for their own health, but this cannot be done by edict. It needs education and support, which requires investment.

There clearly needs to be a public debate about the boundaries of care. I have stated repeatedly in this book that the battle between infinite demand and finite resources cannot end well. Offering infinite resources is impossible – other than in the very short term, as was seen in the acute phase of the Covid-19 pandemic – so a clear vision of what healthcare should offer must be clearly defined. Is the challenge of being universal, high-quality and comprehensive unachievable? It would be intolerable and unethical to accept anything that was not high-quality and I'm a firm believer in the moral imperative of offering a universal system, so this leaves the comprehensive offer as the key area to be debated. Should there be limits on what is offered? And how have we reached a situation where healthcare is the default solution for so many of society's challenges?

In Chapter 1, I wrote about the pharmaceutical industry researching a medication to treat loneliness. While this example of a medical solution for a non-medical problem may be extreme, it perfectly demonstrates the porous boundaries of healthcare. The British prime minister Boris Johnson's statement that general practitioners would be able to *prescribe* cycling as an aid to fitness and weight loss is a classic example of the gradual medicalization of everyday life.[5]

By focusing on non-medical solutions, the benefits can not only be greater but dramatically cheaper – as well as more humane. Take the example of the small Somerset town of Frome, which I mentioned briefly in Chapter 9.

Back in 2013, Dr Helen Kingston, a local GP concerned about the number of patients who were unhappy with the medicalization of their lives, launched a project called Compassionate Frome.[6] Frome Medical Practice combined a compassionate programme of community development with routine medical care. They recognized that the impact of social connectedness can be greater than giving up smoking, reducing excessive drinking, reducing obesity and any other preventative interventions. In particular, they became aware of the role played by primary and community services in identifying those people who are in need of support at moments of crisis. Care coordination teams systematically enabled these people to be offered the help they needed.

Remarkably, when isolated people with health problems were supported by community groups and volunteers, the number of emergency admissions to hospital decreased spectacularly. The number of admissions per 1,000 population in Frome fell from twenty-five to twenty-one, at a time when for Somerset as a whole it increased from 27.8 to 35.7.[7]

But as the focus of this book has been the affordability of healthcare, we should also take note of the savings. The cost of unplanned hospital admissions in Frome fell from £5.7 million in 2013–2014 to £4.5 million in 2016–2017, a reduction of 20.8 per cent.

The Compassionate Communities model has three main components.

1. Through making the most of the supportive networks of family, friends and neighbours, people build care and connectedness, sharing companionship and values.
2. Building networks of support for the routine aspects of life, such as shopping, cooking, cleaning and providing lifts.
3. Linking to community activity, such as choirs, walking groups and other interest groups where people can make friendships.

The idea behind the project is straightforward and humane. It aims to reduce isolation and loneliness in what is frequently a disconnected society, while significantly reducing healthcare costs. Kindness, compassion and community gets better results than focusing only on the medical model.

There are biochemical reasons why community engagement diminishes inflammation, and why inflammation causes ill health. So much of our research has been on cure – and as someone who has survived cancer, I'm very grateful. But we need to put much more energy into understanding and supporting care, while also improving the quality of life in every age group. Yet again, this means ensuring that public health, general practice and community care are right at the top of our priorities rather than languishing at the bottom.

This need for a different approach impacts on medicine worldwide. In a remarkable paper entitled 'How American Medicine Is Destroying Itself', Daniel Callahan and Sherwin B. Nuland wrote:

> Among the elderly, the struggle against disease has begun to look like the trench warfare of World War I: little real progress in taking enemy territory but enormous economic and human cost in trying to do so. Our main achievements today consist of devising ways to marginally extend the lives of the very sick … Ours is now a medicine that may doom most of us to an old age that will end badly: with our declining bodies falling apart as they always have but devilishly – and expensively – stretching out the suffering and decay.[8]

So what's to be done? I do not claim to have all the answers, though I hope I've asked some of the right questions. Nevertheless, there are many issues that could be tackled.

If it doesn't work, don't do it

In Chapter 4, I wrote about Atul Gawande's 2009 report on the remarkable variability in healthcare costs between comparable populations in the US.[9] His conclusion was stark: the primary cause of extreme costs was the overuse of medicine. Many procedures were being done unnecessarily, and only the doctors' bank accounts were benefitting.

This phenomenon exists all around the world. It is not necessarily driven by greed, but it often occurs when doctors don't realize that a procedure is less valuable than they think. In my own early days in medicine, I used some treatments with the best of intentions – treatments that have since been shown to be entirely useless, or even dangerous.

As a result, a number of organizations around the world have attempted to develop lists of healthcare procedures that are of little or no value to the patient. One study in the Netherlands examined 193 clinical guidelines and found a total of 1,366 lower-value services.[10] The majority (77 per cent) of them referred to care that should not be offered at all, whereas 23 per cent recommended aspects of care that should not be offered routinely.

In the UK, NICE has also made a significant number of similar recommendations.[11,12] A review of them by the Academy of Medical Royal Colleges stated that doctors have an ethical duty to prevent waste in the NHS; the savings of nearly £2 billion could be used more effectively elsewhere.[13] Can you think of any logical reason why any doctor should continue to use therapies that have been proven to have no value? Neither can I, which brings us to the next solution.

Tackling waste

In Chapter 1, I described a 2019 report that concluded that about $1 of every $4 spent on healthcare in the United States may be wasted due to a combination of avoidable administrative hassles, failures in coordination and delivery of services, use of unnecessary treatments and fraud.[14] The total annual cost of waste in the US healthcare system has been estimated at between $760 billion and $935 billion.

A 2017 OECD report titled 'Tackling Wasteful Spending on Health' showed that the cost of administering health systems on average represents 3 per cent of all health spending but varies massively between countries, with no obvious correlation with performance.[15] As the report made clear, it is never easy to acknowledge ineffective spending, but opportunities exist to deliver better-value care. Cutting waste will produce significant savings, and such opportunities must be pursued by policymakers struggling to cope with increasing healthcare expenditure.

In England, a report on waste in non-specialist acute hospitals in the NHS showed about £5 billion of unwanted variation in costs.[16] The report made fifteen recommendations designed to tackle this problem and help trusts match the best. As an example, the average price paid for a hip prosthesis varied between £788 and £1,590, with the hospitals that bought the most tending not to pay the lowest price. Other initiatives that could be replicated in every healthcare system include 'Getting it Right First Time', a programme designed to tackle variations in the way services are delivered across the NHS and to share best practice.[17]

Tackling waste also means tackling duplication, which wastes time for patients and clinicians, as well as resources. On a simple level, the absurd situation whereby a patient sometimes needs one appointment for a consultation, another for a blood test, another for an X-ray and another to get the results takes up a remarkable amount of time and resource. A Spanish study in 2019 that looked at the impact of re-engineering outpatient processes using a patient-centred approach showed that productivity increased by 34 per cent, satisfaction improved and complaints fell.[18]

The potential for community diagnostic hubs (or NHS 'one-stop shops') in terms of reducing duplication and wasted patient time is significant. While a patient-centred approach to improving efficiency can pay real dividends, pursuing efficiency too far can be detrimental – as was clear in the English NHS when the coronavirus pandemic revealed the underlying lack of capacity in hospitals. Reducing the number of empty beds in any hospital can seem like a logical approach, but there needs to be capacity to deal with peaks of demand. It is a false economy to cut all services to the bone.

Waste isn't a problem that's restricted to the UK. For instance, the United States typically spends approximately twice as much as any other high-income country on medical care, yet its utilization rates are largely similar. Prices of labour, administrative costs and goods, including pharmaceuticals, appear to be the major drivers of the difference in overall cost. As patients, physicians, policymakers and legislators debate the future of the US healthcare system, such data are needed to inform policy decisions. Talking about cost-effectiveness should never be dismissed as demanding rationing – it is simply being rational.

Excessively expensive therapies

Should the price of therapies be set by the value they bring or by the maximum the market can bear? Organizations like NICE in the UK are well positioned to make decisions about cost-effectiveness. No one, apart from the exceedingly wealthy, chooses to spend money without asking, 'Is this worth the price I'm being asked to pay?' – and there is no reason why healthcare products should be any different.

Organizations such as NICE focus on key criteria including the use of evidence, patient involvement, clinical expertise and transparency in order to make decisions about cost-effectiveness. Keeping such decisions independent of politicians remains critical for public trust. One radical solution would involve the state taking control of the pharmaceutical industry. This suggestion, which is flagged up occasionally by commentators, is too complex and political an issue for this book, but it might well be possible for the state to govern much of the drug innovation process. This would help to control a system that is currently not working to the overall benefit of society.

In the meantime, there is clearly a place for greater transparency around drug pricing. While scrutiny might decrease pricing power, a public debate and the development of trust in the industry might in the longer term produce a more sustainable business model. It is inappropriate for an industry that is literally a matter of life and death to so many people to be so shrouded in secrecy.

However, it is possible to be optimistic about the pharmaceutical industry. It is encouraging that a new generation of leaders believe there is more to the industry than profit. For instance, a new American start-up called EQRx plans to revamp the traditional approach to drug development, launching drugs more quickly and at a lower cost, creating 'novel, patent-protected medicines at prices that are more affordable for people and sustainable for healthcare systems'.[19] Alexis Borisy, the chairman and CEO of EQRx, has been quoted as saying that drastic action is needed as the price of new medicines is 'pushing beyond the limits of common sense, preventing people and society from equally benefiting from innovation'. Sadly, these views are not yet typical.

The boundaries of funded healthcare
In the UK, ever since the NHS was founded in 1948, there has been a gradual dilution of the universal offer of free care of everything for

everyone. Most patients over the age of sixteen and under the age of sixty, for instance, contribute to the cost of their prescription drugs.

If providing everything for everyone is becoming challenging, society needs to debate whether there are aspects of care that should no longer be part of the all-inclusive offer. One logical and effective model that would facilitate such a discussion is a citizens' assembly. The people who would be chosen to take part would be reflective of the wider population, both in terms of demographics and attitudes. Such assemblies have been used around the world, with particular success in Ireland – where they debated and made recommendations that changed the abortion law – and in Canada. Wherever they are used, participants are asked to make trade-offs and arrive at workable recommendations. The citizens' council of NICE, which was set up in the early days of the organization, provided a public perspective on moral and ethical issues when producing guidance and decisions.

Determining the boundaries of care requires political courage, and they will need to be kept up to date following new research and discoveries. But without some form of decision-making process, new areas of provision will continue to be driven by the pharmaceutical industry, whose motivation might be determined more by their own self-interest.

Every country's healthcare system will need to address this challenge. Even systems that are funded through insurance rather than taxation will require clarity of purpose – after all, funds are never infinite, however they are generated. If this seems too difficult, the alternative is to leave such decisions to be dictated by commercial pressures. Should the healthcare system feel that it is obliged to offer treatment for every new condition proposed by pharmaceutical or healthcare tech companies, or should there be some form of prioritization? Of course, if there turns out to be sufficient funding to provide everything for everyone, I will be delighted to have been proven wrong – and more than a little astonished.

There is one additional challenge that requires debate. In systems that provide universal health coverage for all citizens, should there be any obligations on the individual? For instance, some people believe that an obese citizen who doesn't exercise, uses alcohol to excess and has an appetite for recreational drugs should not be entitled to state-funded healthcare. Equally, there are others who argue strongly that such an individual may well be responding to a disadvantaged upbringing and may be more deserving than most. Such debates are challenging and complex, but they should not be ignored.

During the Covid-19 pandemic, we saw how the choice by some citizens not to be vaccinated ultimately impacted on the care of others. If an intensive care bed was taken by someone who had declined vaccination and surgery for another patient with a non-Covid condition was delayed or cancelled as a result, this illustrated perfectly the dilemma. As John Donne wrote over four hundred years ago, 'No man is an island, entire of itself'. Our individual behaviours and choices massively impact on others. It raises the question of whether we are a 'me society' or a 'we society'.

Choosing wisely
When people are faced with a healthcare challenge, non-medical approaches can often be superior – as illustrated by the use of community activity to improve quality of life in Frome, while reducing healthcare costs. 'Choosing Wisely' is a major international campaign that engages physicians and patients in conversations about unnecessary tests, treatments and procedures. It was created

to challenge the idea that doing more is better, promoting the idea that 'just because we can doesn't always mean we should'.

The campaign encourages patients to ask their doctors and nurses four questions:

1. What are the benefits?
2. What are the risks?
3. What are the alternatives?
4. What if I do nothing?

The Choosing Wisely campaign began in the US in 2012, where more than sixty medical societies created lists of tests, treatments or procedures where there is scientific evidence that they are either not beneficial or even cause harm. A website offers advice for clinicians and patients, particularly concerning commonly used procedures that may be ineffective. Concerns that campaigns like this are overly focused on cost are entirely illogical – after all, you are not being deprived if you don't have a test that doesn't benefit you in any way. If being treated logically saves money, that is a positive side effect. And sadly, not all doctors are as well informed as they might be. A 2007 paper in the *Journal of the American Medical Association* found that it took ten years for much of the medical community to stop referencing popular practices after their efficacy was scientifically disproven.[20]

Choosing Wisely has spread internationally. It launched in Canada in 2014, after which Italy adopted the same principles in a campaign called 'Doing More Does not Mean Doing Better'. Numerous other countries, including the Netherlands, England, Japan, Australia, New Zealand, Germany, Italy, Switzerland, Wales, Scotland and Denmark, have also launched similar campaigns.

The recognition that doctors and other clinicians often carry out work that is neither necessary nor beneficial is intriguing. Many doctors argue that their treatment choices are to some extent determined by their patients' expectations rather than what is necessary. When doctors are patients themselves, the treatments they choose are frequently different from those they typically offer to patients. In a study in the *Archives of Internal Medicine*, a group of doctors received a survey that either asked them to assume they were the patient suffering from bowel cancer or asked them about the advice they gave to others.[21] Of the physicians who answered for themselves, 38 per cent chose a treatment that carried a higher risk of death but fewer side effects; only a quarter said they would recommend that treatment to their patients.

We have an intriguing scenario where doctors seem to second-guess what their patients want, often without good evidence. This has profound connotations; a King's Fund report asked whether we're wasting money on care that patients don't in fact want.[22]

In 'Patients' Preferences Matter', Professor Al Mulley looked at areas of medical practice where fully informed patients are less likely to choose surgery. I know from my own career that when I discussed options with patients, they would often end up asking me what I advised. In retrospect, I suspect I would jump to my own conclusion without finding out what really mattered to them – what Al Mulley describes as a 'preference misdiagnosis'. As the report says:

> Many doctors aspire to excellence in diagnosing disease. Far fewer, unfortunately, aspire to the same standards of excellence in diagnosing what patients want. In fact … preference misdiagnoses are commonplace. In part, this is because doctors are rarely made aware that they

have made a preference misdiagnosis. It is the silent misdiagnosis.

Finding out patients' genuine wishes can benefit them hugely. Furthermore, as an unintended consequence of the preference of fully informed patients to choose fewer treatments, the NHS would likely save billions of pounds. Vast numbers of prescriptions, investigations and operations may have been carried out because doctors assumed they were what their patients wanted. To make the situation even more complex, patients will have been grateful for care that they probably didn't need; while they might think 'the doctor wouldn't recommend it if it wasn't necessary', the doctors might be choosing a treatment 'because that's what my patient wanted'. This state of confusion would not be out of place in *Alice in Wonderland*.

Ensuring that patients understand the risks and the benefits of a given course of action can make an immense difference to the quality, quantity and cost of healthcare. It would help immensely if clinical trials focused on the issues that are of most interest to patients rather than prioritizing the interest of researchers. However, I am encouraged by developments such as the Personalised Care Institute, which has been set up to equip health and care professionals with the knowledge, skills and confidence to involve patients in decisions about their care. As I described earlier, evidence shows that this leads to better health outcomes and increased patient and clinician satisfaction; it is both a major practical change to the NHS and a key part of the NHS Long Term Plan. If we can integrate healthcare services around the individual, it will be a major step forward.

Curing and caring

For a long time, it seemed that medical advances were potentially unlimited, that we could take on and defeat one condition after another. After all, medical science had successfully eradicated smallpox and was making good progress in tackling many of the other major infectious diseases. It seemed to many people that developments such as genomics, stem-cell technology, personalized medicines and early prevention would result in us all living long and healthy lives, followed by rapid deterioration and death at an advanced age – an aspiration that seems as far away as ever. Every small medical advance has massive economic and human cost, and ill health appears to have infinite reinforcements.

We are all going to die. While it is wonderful that medical science is able to spend unimaginable sums researching and treating disease, we seem to have forgotten than death is not the worst thing that can happen to the elderly. Disability, loneliness, isolation, frailty, poverty and fear can make their last months – if not years – something dreadful, and yet we spend nowhere near as much time or money trying to address these issues.

A letter to *The Times* from a palliative medicine consultant movingly focused on another aspect of end-of-life care. He wrote,

> A significant proportion of my time as a senior hospital palliative medicine consultant is spent advising medical and surgical colleagues in hospital to withdraw or stop inappropriate investigations and futile treatments that prolong a patient's suffering without adding any dignity or quality to life. This is called good medical practice. I get increasingly frustrated when I see terminally ill

patients who are in their last weeks or days of life being kept in hospital and overtreated. Because we can treat a medical condition does not equate to having to treat it.[23]

This final phrase is so true in so many aspects of medicine.

Our healthcare systems must have a culture of care rather than a near total focus on cure, including more support to allow the elderly to live independently in their own homes. Some of us may die earlier, but we will live more fulfilled lives and will hopefully have better deaths. We are currently using a twentieth-century model of hospital-based service delivery to meet twenty-first-century needs.

As Lord Nigel Crisp has written, 'A transition is underway around the world from hospital- and illness-based systems to person- and health-based ones, where, aided by technology, more services are provided in communities and homes.'[24] Sadly, where there are funding pressures, it is the social and community services that are cut, not least because of the public outcry that follows any threat to a local hospital. In stark contrast, cuts to community services such as district nursing rarely make the news. It is not just policymakers and clinicians who need to understand the need for change – it is all of us.

Caring for patients is clearly a fundamental role of any healthcare organization. Sadly, over the past decades, many aspects of healthcare delivery have been industrialized, with clinicians learning to 'process' patients while focusing on efficiency. In his challenging and inspirational book *Why We Revolt*, Victor Montori encouraged healthcare organizations to turn away from this industrialized focus towards a greater focus on caring and kindness, looking at the world through the eyes of the individual patient. As a seemingly trivial example – which actually speaks volumes – the all-too-prevalent block booking of a group of patients who are all given outpatient appointments at exactly the same time, and which inevitably results in almost all of them waiting, is thoughtless and prioritizes the system over the individual. To offer a more personalized system isn't just kinder; it reduces stress and hassle across the whole team. Having kinder, more patient-centred values isn't to deny patients the potential benefits of modern medicine. Indeed, blending a kinder and more human approach with the best that science can offer is the best of both worlds. This isn't just better for patients – it is far more satisfying for clinicians too. It will be fascinating to follow pilot studies that explore this way of working.[25]

Aspirations

There can be little doubt that healthcare is on the cusp of great change. Astonishing advances in personalized therapies, genomics, big data and artificial intelligence will have an impact, but this won't come for free.

We need to be clear what the focus of healthcare should be. While the benefits of scientific and technical research are huge, we should not ignore the importance of care. We must put as much effort into the war on frailty and loneliness as we do into the war on cancer. We need to ensure that we have a workforce that can offer continuity of care whenever it is appropriate – after all, it is associated with reduced mortality, greater patient satisfaction, better health promotion, increased adherence to medication and less hospital usage.[26]

One unintended side effect of many recent healthcare policies has been a reduction in continuity of care. As Professor Martin Marshall, chair of the Royal College of General Practitioners, has said:

> It feels to me that the relationship between a patient and their GP is as important as a scalpel is to a surgeon. If relationships were a drug, NICE and other guideline developers would have to mandate their use. But relationships, and the ways in which we build and utilize them, aren't drugs, so we don't talk about them very much.[27]

Indeed, over the past decades, the UK has invested billions of pounds in new drugs. While some have been immensely worthwhile, others have added little of value. At precisely the same time, underinvestment in the healthcare workforce has had a massive impact on the ability of citizens to be able to build up a trusting relationship with a clinician. Continuity of care is increasingly rare, and yet we know that it offers true and major benefits. A trusting relationship with a clinician has been proven to improve patient experience and outcomes, while also reducing mortality. It is one of the most effective interventions we know for multimorbidity. It reduces emergency department attendance, hospital admissions and overall healthcare costs.

As patients have to navigate the complexity of modern healthcare, the vast amount of information available online and the increasing advances in technology, many will need a trusted interpreter to help them find the best solutions that work for them. This partnership approach to healthcare, with clinicians focusing on individuals, will be increasingly important.[28] Clinicians will work in partnership with technology rather than being replaced or feeling threatened by it.

And these benefits can work both ways. Having an ongoing relationship with patients is much more satisfying for clinicians; it boosts morale and reduces the likelihood that doctors and nurses will leave healthcare or retire early. If a drug this effective, and with so many benefits, was denied to the public, there would be an outcry.

It's all very puzzling. This gradual diminution of the doctor, patient relationship is an unintended side effect of a raft of different policies. A generation ago, most people would talk of 'my doctor'. Today, at a time when a trusting relationship with an expert clinician has never been more important, it has never been more endangered.

In a world where many more of us will develop multiple health problems, we must encourage more young doctors to become generalists, to be supported by specialists when needed. We need to support the introduction of truly personalized care, in which people have both choice and control over the way their care is planned and delivered, and which is based on what matters to them and their individual strengths and needs.[29] We have to recognize that costs are escalating in every healthcare system in the world, however they are organized. But despite this, more people are suffering poor health, declining ability and reduced mobility in their later years, meaning they are spending greater proportions of their lives in consulting rooms or hospitals. Is that really what we're trying to achieve?

We need to tackle waste, duplication of effort, poor end-of-life care and a deterioration in doctor–patient relationships. We need to focus on prevention. The inverse care law must be not only understood, but tackled. The profit motive cannot be the only thing that is allowed to drive pharmaceutical companies. There are good people out there, after all, and they can make a huge difference.

Most of all, we must remember that healthcare is a human business. Kindness, humanity and caring really matter – and they don't need to cost anything.

Acknowledgements

This book is the result of a lifetime spent in medicine, listening, learning, watching and discussing. The opinions expressed are entirely mine and in no way necessarily represent the views of any of the multiplicity of organizations I have worked in and with.

While writing this book I had particular support and advice from Stuart Nuttall, Nish Manek, Jane Gizbert, Richard Taunt, David Whitrap, Helen Kingston and Andrew Grey – though any errors are entirely my responsibility. I am most grateful to them, and also to Sam Hodder, my agent at Blake Friedmann, Nick Humphrey, my editor, and all the team at Atlantic Books for their encouragement and tolerance while personal and global events impacted on the timeframe of this book.

I learned almost everything I know about healthcare from my patients and from my colleagues. I can't even begin to list all the inspirational and exceptional people that I've been lucky enough to meet, at least not without doubling the length of this book. But thank you to all of you, and particularly to all the staff in the National Health Service who treated my cancer and cared for me over the past couple of years. They taught me a lot, too.

Finally, my wife Barbara has been a huge support throughout my whole career, from my earliest days as a student, all the way through to encouraging me while writing this book. I couldn't have done it without her.

Endnotes

Foreword

1. 'Prime Minister's Statement on Coronavirus (COVID-19)', 17 March 2020, https://www.gov.uk/government/speeches/pm-statement-on-coronavirus-17-march-2020
2. 'Where Are the Ventilators?: Cuomo Pleads for More Help for New York', *New York Times*, 24 March 2020, https://www.nytimes.com/video/us/politics/100000007051271/cuomo-coronavirus-update.html
3. Office for National Statistics, https://www.ons.gov.uk/peoplepopulationandcommunity/healthandsocialcare/healthcaresystem/articles/howdoesukhealthcarespendingcomparewithothercountries/2019-08-29
4. R. McNair Wilson, *The Beloved Physician*, John Murray, 1926
5. 'NHS Pressures in England: Waiting Times, Demand and Capacity', 17 December 2019, https://commonslibrary.parliament.uk/nhs-pressures-in-england-waiting-times-demand-and-capacity/
6. 'LSE–*Lancet* Commission on the Future of the NHS: Re-laying the Foundations for an Equitable and Efficient Health and Care Service after COVID-19', 6 May 2021, https://doi.org/10.1016/S0140-6736(21)00232-4
7. 'An Initial Response to the Prime Minister's Announcement on Health, Social Care and National Insurance', 7 September 2021, https://ifs.org.uk/publications/15597

Chapter 1: We've Got a Problem

1. 'Coronavirus: ExCeL Centre Planned as NHS Field Hospital', BBC News, 24 March 2020, https://www.bbc.co.uk/news/health-52018477
2. 'Revealed: What Really Happened In The Nightingales', *Huffington Post*, 29 March 2021, https://www.huffingtonpost.co.uk/entry/nightingale-hospitals-covid-patient-numbers_uk_605a0dd6c5b6cebf58d220eb

ENDNOTES

3 Public Spending on Health: A Closer Look at Global Trends, World Health Organization, April 2018, https://apps.who.int/iris/rest/bitstreams/1165184/retrieve

4 'Levelling Up Health, All Party Parliamentary Group for Longevity', April 2021, https://static1.squarespace.com/static/5d349e15bf59a30001efeaeb/t/606f7115c96b9c377aa2e3bc/1617916190582/Levelling+up+Health+Report+9+April+2021+FINAL.pdf

5 J.T. Chen, N. Krieger, 'Revealing the Unequal Burden of COVID-19 by Income, Race/Ethnicity and Household Crowding: US County vs. ZIP Code Analyses', Harvard Center for Population and Development Studies, 21 April 2020, https://cdn1.sph.harvard.edu/wp-content/uploads/sites/1266/2020/04/HCPDS_Volume-19_No_1_20_covid19_RevealingUnequalBurden_HCPDSWorkingPaper_04212020-1.pdf

6 'Mapa interactiu de casos per ABS', Generalitat de Catalunya, https://aquas.gencat.cat/ca/actualitat/ultimes-dades-coronavirus/mapa-per-abs/

7 The Burden of COVID-19 in Brazil is Greater in Areas with High Social Deprivation', *Journal of Travel Medicine*, Volume 27, Issue 7, October 2020, https://doi.org/10.1093/jtm/taaa145

8 'Socio-demographic Risk Factors of COVID-19 Deaths in Sweden: A Nationwide Register Study', Stockholm University Demography Unit, 11 September 2020, https://su.figshare.com/articles/preprint/Socio-demographic_risk_factors_of_COVID-19_deaths_in_Sweden_A_nationwide_register_study/12420347

9 https://committees.parliament.uk/oralevidence/1588/html/

10 'National Life Tables – Life Expectancy in the UK: 2018 to 2020', Office for National Statistics, 23 September 2021, https://www.ons.gov.uk/peoplepopulationandcommunity/birthsdeathsandmarriages/lifeexpectancies/bulletins/nationallifetablesunitedkingdom/2018to2020

11 '83% of People with Cancer Face Financial Hit, Charity Says', *Independent*, 7 December 2021, https://www.independent.ie/world-news/83-of-people-with-cancer-face-financial-hit-charity-says-41128886.html

12 'Scientists Are Working on a Pill for Loneliness', *Guardian*, 26 January 2019, https://www.theguardian.com/us-news/2019/jan/26/pill-for-loneliness-psychology-science-medicine

13 'Doctors to Prescribe Bike Rides to Tackle UK Obesity Crisis', *Guardian*, 26 July 2020, https://www.theguardian.com/politics/2020/jul/26/doctors-to-prescribe-bike-rides-to-tackle-uk-obesity-crisis-amid-coronavirus-risk

14 E. Yong, 'How the Pandemic Defeated America', *The Atlantic*, 4 August 2020, https://www.theatlantic.com/magazine/archive/2020/09/coronavirus-american-failure/614191

ENDNOTES

15 'Drug Costing £10 Million Per Patient to Become Most Expensive Treatment on the NHS', *Daily Telegraph,* 28 January 2015, https://www.telegraph.co.uk/news/nhs/11373509/Drug-costing-10-million-per-patient-to-become-most-expensive-treatment-on-the-NHS.html

16 'This New Treatment Could Save the Lives of Babies. But It Costs $2.1 Million', *New York Times,* 24 May 2019

17 'NHS England strikes deal on life-saving gene-therapy drug that can help babies with rare genetic disease move and walk', NHS England, 8 March 2021, https://www.england.nhs.uk/2021/03/nhs-england-strikes-deal-on-life-saving-gene-therapy-drug-that-can-help-babies-with-rare-genetic-disease-move-and-walk/

18 How is the NHS Performing? December 2018 Quarterly Monitoring Report, The King's Fund, 21 December 2018, https://www.kingsfund.org.uk/publications/how-nhs-performing-december-2018

19 W. Shrank, T. Rogstad, N. Parekh, 'Waste in the US Health Care System: Estimated Costs and Potential for Savings', *JAMA,* 2019;322(15):1501-1509, https://jamanetwork.com/journals/jama/article-abstract/2752664

20 I. Scott, S. Duckett, 'In Search of Professional Consensus in Defining and Reducing Low-Value Care', *Medical Journal of Australia,* 17 August 2015, 17;203(4):179–81, https://www.ncbi.nlm.nih.gov/pubmed/26268286?dopt=Abstract

21 'Facts and figures on the NHS at 70', Nuffield Trust, July 2018, https://www.nuffieldtrust.org.uk/files/2018-07/facts-and-figs-website.pdf

22 'Spending on Health and Social Care over the Next 50 Years: Why Think Long Term?' The King's Fund, 31 January 2013, https://www.kingsfund.org.uk/publications/spending-health-and-social-care-over-next-50-years

23 'The Long-Term Outlook for Health Care Spending', Congress of the United States Congressional Budget Office, November 2007, https://www.cbo.gov/sites/default/files/110th-congress-2007-2008/reports/11-13-lt-health.pdf

24 'Trends in Future Health Financing and Coverage: Future Health Spending and Universal Health Coverage in 188 countries, 2016–40', *The Lancet,* 17 April 2018, https://www.thelancet.com/journals/lancet/article/PIIS0140-6736(18)30697-4/fulltext

25 'Even Insured Can Face Crushing Medical Debt, Study Finds', *New York Times,* 5 January 2015, https://www.nytimes.com/2016/01/06/upshot/lost-jobs-houses-savings-even-insured-often-face-crushing-medical-debt.html

26 'Average Health Care Costs and Ways to Save', *The Balance,* 24 December 2021, https://www.thebalance.com/healthcare-costs-3306068

27 'The Rising Cost of Medicines to the NHS: What's the Story?', The King's Fund, 26 April 2018, https://www.kingsfund.org.uk/publications/rising-cost-medicines-nhs

ENDNOTES

28 'Health Economics: The Cancer Drugs Cost Conundrum', Cancer Research, 10 August 2016, http://www.cancerresearchuk.org/funding-for-researchers/research-features/2016-08-10-health-economics-the-cancer-drugs-cost-conundrum

29 K. Arrow, 'Uncertainty and the Welfare Economics of Medical Care', *The American Economic Review*, Vol. 53, No. 5 (December 1963), pp. 941–973, https://www.jstor.org/stable/1812044?seq=1#page_scan_tab_contents

30 'One Child, a $21-Million Medical Bill: How a Tiny Number of Patients Poses a Huge Challenge for Medi-Cal', *LA Times*, 16 July 2017, http://www.latimes.com/politics/la-me-21-million-patient-20170716-story.html

31 'Ulana Suprun: The Accidental Reformer', *The Lancet*, 1 September 2018, https://doi.org/10.1016/S0140-6736(18)31855-5

32 'COVID-19 Highlights Urgent Need to Reboot Global Effort to End Tuberculosis', World Health Organization, 22 March 2021, https://www.who.int/news/item/22-03-2021-covid-19-highlights-urgent-need-to-reboot-global-effort-to-end-tuberculosis

33 R. Dobos, *Mirage of Health: Utopias, Progress, and Biological Change*, Harper & Row, 1959

Chapter 2: How Did We Get Here?

1 'What Is Happening to Life Expectancy in England?', The King's Fund, 6 December 2021, https://www.kingsfund.org.uk/publications/whats-happening-life-expectancy-england

2 '63,000 Extra Deaths and a Year Off Life Expectancy: COVID in 2020 in England & Wales', University of Oxford, 27 January 2021, https://www.ox.ac.uk/news/2021-01-27-63000-extra-deaths-and-year-life-expectancy-covid-2020-england-wales

3 'Tube Map Used to Plot Londoners' Life Expectancy', BBC News, 20 July 2012, https://www.bbc.co.uk/news/uk-england-london-18917932

4 R. Chetty, M. Stepner, S. Abraham, 'The Association Between Income and Life Expectancy in the United States, 2001–2014', *JAMA*, 2016;315(16):1750–1766, https://jamanetwork.com/journals/jama/article-abstract/2513561

5 'Deaths Involving COVID-19 by Local Area and Socioeconomic Deprivation: Deaths Occurring Between 1 March and 17 April 2020', Office for National Statistics, 1 May 2020. https://www.ons.gov.uk/peoplepopulationandcommunity/birthsdeathsandmarriages/deaths/bulletins/deathsinvolvingcovid19bylocalareasanddeprivation/deathsoccurringbetween1marchand17april

6 'Covid-19 Kills People in the Most Deprived Areas at Double the Rate of Those in the Most Affluent', Nuffield Trust, 6 May 2020, https://www.

ENDNOTES

nuffieldtrust.org.uk/resource/chart-of-the-week-Covid-19-kills-the-most-deprived-at-double-the-rate-of-affluent-people-like-other-conditions

7 UCL Institute of Health Inequality, http://www.instituteofhealthequity.org/home

8 'Build Back Fairer in Greater Manchester: Health Equity and Dignified Lives', UCL Institute of Health Inequality, June 2021, https://www.instituteofhealthequity.org/resources-reports/build-back-fairer-in-greater-manchester-health-equity-and-dignified-lives

9 'Measles Jab Saves over 20 Million Young Lives in 15 years, but Hundreds of Children Still Die of the Disease Every Day', UNICEF, 10 November 2016, https://www.unicef.org/eca/press-releases/measles-jab-saves-million-young-lives

10 'Facts and FAQ About Down Syndrome', Global Down Syndrome Foundation, https://www.globaldownsyndrome.org/about-down-syndrome/facts-about-down-syndrome/

11 'Twice as Long – Life Expectancy Around the World', Our World in Data, 8 October 2018, https://ourworldindata.org/life-expectancy-globally

12 'Global Food Prices Drop to a Five-Year Low', The World Bank, 1 July 2015, http://www.worldbank.org/en/news/press-release/2015/07/01/global-food-prices-drop-to-a-five-year-low

13 'Food Price Deflation Cheers Consumers, Hurts Farmers, Grocers and Restaurants', *Wall Street Journal*, 29 August 2016, https://www.wsj.com/articles/food-price-deflation-cheers-consumers-hurts-farmers-grocers-and-restaurants-1472490823

14 'Stroke', National Institute for Health and Care Excellence, https://bnf.nice.org.uk/treatment-summary/stroke.html

15 'Confirmed Impacts: Driving Improvements in NHS Stroke Care', National Audit Office, https://www.nao.org.uk/report/confirmed-impacts-driving-improvements-in-nhs-stroke-care/

16 A. Johnson, 'Proximal Gastric Vagotomy: Does It Have a Place in the Future Management of Peptic Ulcer?', *World Journal of Surgery*, 24, 259–263, 2000, doi: 10.1007, http://citeseerx.ist.psu.edu/viewdoc/download?doi=10.1.1.606.1378&rep=rep1&type=pdf

17 From 'Soundbites', *British Medical Journal*, 12 December 1998, https://www.ncbi.nlm.nih.gov/pmc/articles/PMC1114464/

18 http://www.fph.org.uk/uploads/r_chronology_of_state_medicine.pdf

19 R. McNair Wilson, *The Beloved Physician*, 1926

20 'Trends in Coronary Heart Disease, 1961–2011', British Heart Foundation, https://www.bhf.org.uk/~/media/files/.../bhf-trends-in-coronary-heart-disease.pdf

ENDNOTES

21 'Heart Disease and Stroke Statistics – 2017 Update', A Report From the American Heart Association, 25 January 2017
22 'US Heart Disease Rates Decline', Reuters, 21 March 2016, https://www.reuters.com/article/us-health-heartdisease-us-trends/u-s-heart-disease-rates-decline-idUSKCN0WN2A6
23 J. Tudor Hart, 'The Inverse Care Law', *The Lancet*, 297: 4412, 1971
24 https://doi.org/10.3399/bjgp18X699893
25 D. Sanghavi, 'The History of Cardiac Care: Overtreatment or Impressive Gains?', *The Lancet*, 31 August 2013, https://doi.org/10.1016/S0140-6736(13)61727-4
26 http://justageing.equalityhumanrights.com/wp-content/uploads/2009/09/The-future-of-ageing.pdf
27 E. Wallace, C. Salisbury, B. Guthrie et al, 'Managing patients with multimorbidity in primary care, *British Medical Journal*, 350:h176, 2015.
28 'Delivering Better Services for People with Long-Term Conditions', The King's Fund, October 2013, https://www.kingsfund.org.uk/sites/default/files/field/field_publication_file/delivering-better-services-for-people-with-long-term-conditions.pdf
29 K, Barnett, S. Mercer, M. Norbury, G. Watt, S. Wyke and B. Guthrie, 'Epidemiology of Multimorbidity and Implications for Health Care, Research and Medical Education: A Cross-Sectional Study', *The Lancet*, 7 July 2012, https://www.ncbi.nlm.nih.gov/pubmed/22579043
30 K. Nicholson et al, 'Prevalence, Characteristics and Patterns of Patients with Multimorbidity in Primary Care: A Retrospective Cohort Analysis in Canada', *British Journal of General Practice*, September 2019, p. 439
31 'Future Hospital Commission', Royal College of Physicians, 16 September 2013, https://www.rcplondon.ac.uk/projects/outputs/future-hospital-commission
32 'The Future Doctor Programme', Health Education England,Paying the Price https://www.hee.nhs.uk/sites/default/files/documents/Future%20Doctor%20Co-Created%20Vision%20-%20FINAL%20%28typo%20corrected%29.pdf
33 N. Timmins, *The Five Giants: A Biography of the Welfare State*, Harper Collins, p. 267
34 K. Amadeo, 'The Rising Cost of Health Care by Year and Its Causes', *The Balance,* 26 March 2021, https://www.thebalance.com/causes-of-rising-healthcare-costs-4064878
35 'Public Expenditure Statistical Analysis 2017', HM Treasury
36 'OECD Health Data', *OECD Health Statist*ics, doi: 10.1787/data-00350-en
37 https://www.who.int/whr/2008/whr08_en.pdf

ENDNOTES

38 H. Sandvik, O. Hetlevik, J. Blinkenberg and S. Hunskaar, 'Continuity in General Practice as Predictor of Mortality, Acute Hospitalisation and Use of Out-of-Hours Care: A Registry-Based Observational Study in Norway', *British Journal of General Practice*, doi: https://doi.org/10.3399/BJGP.2021.0340

Chapter 3: Paying the Price

1 'How Much Does an MRI Machine Cost?', LBN Medical, https://lbnmedical.com/how-much-does-an-mri-machine-cost/
2 D. Fletcher et al, 'Improving Theatre Turnaround Time', *BMJ Quality Improvement Programme,* http://bmjopenquality.bmj.com/content/6/1/u219831.w8131#ref-2
3 'Average Costs of a New Hip Prosthesis in Selected Countries in 2013 (in US Dollars)', Statista, https://www.statista.com/statistics/312251/average-cost-of-hip-prosthesis-by-country/
4 http://www.ifhp.com/insights/ifhp-comparative-price-report-issued/
5 'How Much Does Hip Replacement Cost?', Cost Helper Health, http://health.costhelper.com/hip-replacement.html
6 'The Cost of Hip Replacement Surgery in Australia: A Closer Look into the Actual Cost for Australians Wanting Hip Replacement Surgery', People Pledge Australia Blog, http://peoplepledge.com.au/blog/the-cost-of-hip-replacement-surgery-in-australia-a-closer-look-into-the-actual-cost-for-australians-wanting-hip-replacement-surgery/
7 http://www.who.int/entity/whr/2008/whr08_en.pdf
8 D. Matheson, 'Will Universal Health Coverage (UHC) Lead to the Freedom to Lead Flourishing and Healthy Lives?; Comment on "Inequities in the Freedom to Lead a Flourishing and Healthy Life: Issues for Healthy Public Policy"', *International Journal of Health Policy and Management*, https://www.ijhpm.com/article_2937_616.html
9 http://www.who.int/life-course/news/events/uhc-day/en/
10 'Universal Health Coverage (UHC)', World Health Organization, 1 April 2021, https://www.who.int/en/news-room/fact-sheets/detail/universal-health-coverage-(uhc)
11 Ibid
12 'Universal Health Coverage Key to Safer, Fairer World, Says WHO Chief on Eve of World Health Day', *UN News*, 6 April 2018, https://news.un.org/en/story/2018/04/1006742
13 M.R. Reich et al, '50 Years of Pursuing a Healthy Society in Japan', *The Lancet*, 30 August 2011, https://www.thelancet.com/journals/lancet/article/PIIS0140-6736(11)60274-2/fulltext

ENDNOTES

14 R. Busse et al, 'Statutory Health Insurance in Germany: A Health System Shaped by 135 Years of Solidarity, Self-Governance and Competition', 3 July 2017, https://www.thelancet.com/journals/lancet/article/PIIS0140-6736(17)31280-1/fulltext
15 D. Veksler, 'The One Minute Case Against Socialized Healthcare', One Minute Cases, http://oneminute.rationalmind.net/socialized-healthcare/
16 http://www.nhshistory.net/shorthistory.htm
17 http://www.nationalarchives.gov.uk/cabinetpapers/alevelstudies/origins-nhs.htm
18 *British Medical Journal*, 19 June 1948, p. 1198
19 https://www.sochealth.co.uk/1956/01/10/guillebaud-report/
20 D. Martin et al, 'Canada's Universal Health-Care System: Achieving its Potential', *The Lancet,* 2018;391, pp. 1718–35
21 M. Murray, 'Katrina aid from Cuba? No thanks, says US', NBC News, 12 September 2005, http://www.nbcnews.com/id/9311876/ns/us_news-katrina_the_long_road_back/t/katrina-aid-cuba-no-thanks-says-us
22 B. Bryson, *The Body*, 2019
23 'The Astonishingly High Administrative Costs of US Health Care', *New York Times*, 16 July 2018, https://www.nytimes.com/2018/07/16/upshot/costs-health-care-us.html
24 'Mirror, Mirror 2021: Reflecting Poorly', The Commonwealth Fund, https://www.commonwealthfund.org/publications/fund-reports/2021/aug/mirror-mirror-2021-reflecting-poorly
25 'Current Health Expenditure per Capita, PPP', The World Bank, https://data.worldbank.org/indicator/SH.XPD.CHEX.PP.CD
26 'Brazil's Family Health Programme', *British Medical Journal*, 29 November 2010, https://www.bmj.com/content/341/bmj.c4945
27 A. Shah, 'Health Care Around the World', Global Issues, 22 September 2011, http://www.globalissues.org/article/774/health-care-around-the-world
28 http://www.who.int/nmh/publications/ncd_report2010/en/
29 https://www.who.int/mental_health/prevention/suicide/suicideprevent/en/

Chapter 4: Why Is it All So Expensive?

1 N. Hazra, C. Rudisill and M. Gulliford, 'Determinants of Health Care Costs in the Senior Elderly: Age, Comorbidity, Impairment, or Proximity to Death?', *The European Journal of Health Economics*, 30 August 2017, https://link.springer.com/article/10.1007%2Fs10198-017-0926-2
2 'UK Health Accounts: 2016', Office for National Statistics, 25 April 2018, https://www.ons.gov.uk/peoplepopulationandcommunity/healthandsocialcare/healthcaresystem/bulletins/ukhealthaccounts/2016

ENDNOTES

3 'The NHS Workforce in Numbers', Nuffield Trust, 24 April 2019, https://www.nuffieldtrust.org.uk/resource/the-nhs-workforce-in-numbers

4 'The NHS is the World's Fifth Largest Employer', Nuffield Trust, 27 October 2017, https://www.nuffieldtrust.org.uk/chart/the-nhs-is-the-world-s-fifth-largest-employer

5 https://www.nhsconfed.org/resources/key-statistics-on-the-nhs

6 A. Gawande, 'The Cost Conundrum', *New Yorker*, 1 June 2009

7 https://www.nhs.uk/news/neurology/keyhole-knee-surgery-is-waste-of-time-review-finds/

8 '"Scan because you can", and "boys and toys". Answering the Question of Why We Persist with Low Value Care', *Health Policy*, January 2020, https://www.3vh.org/essential-insights/scan-because-you-can-and-boys-and-toys-answering-the-question-of-why-we-persist-with-low-value-care/

9 B. Hofmann, 'Biases Distorting Priority Setting', *Health Policy*, January 2020, https://doi.org/10.1016/j.healthpol.2019.11.010

10 C. Dyer, 'A New Settlement When Things Go Wrong', *British Medical Journal*, 9 September 2017, p. 348

11 C. Smyth, 'Health Service Faces £77bn Negligence Bill', *The Times*, 14 July 2018, https://www.thetimes.co.uk/edition/news/health-service-faces-77bn-negligence-bill-3trx6qwwt

12 https://resolution.nhs.uk/wp-content/uploads/2017/04/NHS-Resolution-Our-strategy-to-2022-1.pdf

13 R. Ungar, 'The True Cost Of Medical Malpractice – It May Surprise You', *Forbes*, 7 September 2010, https://www.forbes.com/sites/rickungar/2010/09/07/the-true-cost-of-medical-malpractice-it-may-surprise-you/#2e5ec0e52ff5

14 'The Rising Cost of Medicines to the NHS', The King's Fund, https://www.kingsfund.org.uk/sites/default/files/2018-04/Rising-cost-of-medicines.pdf

15 '2018 and Beyond: Outlook and Turning Points', IQVIA, 13 March 2018, https://www.iqvia.com/institute/reports/2018-and-beyond-outlook-and-turning-points

16 M. Duerden, T. Avery, R. Payne, 'Polypharmacy and Medicines Optimisation: Making It Safe and Sound', The King's Fund, 28 November 2013, www.kingsfund.org.uk/publications/polypharmacy-and-medicines-optimisation

17 'National Overprescribing Review Report', https://www.gov.uk/government/publications/national-overprescribing-review-report

18 'Tackling Overprescribing', *British Medical Journal*, 20 October 2021, https://doi.org/10.1136/bmj.n2539

19 'Nearly Half of the UK on Repeat Medication, BGF News, 24 November 2017, https://www.bgf.co.uk/repeat-medication/

ENDNOTES

20 C. Gerry, 'Why Americans Hate Big Pharma More Than Ever', American Council on Science and Health, 9 September 2019, https://www.acsh.org/news/2019/09/09/why-americans-hate-big-pharma-more-ever-14275

21 B. Mole, 'Pfizer CEO Gets 61% Pay Raise – to $27.9 million – as Drug Prices Continue to Climb', Ars Technica, 16 March 2018, https://arstechnica.com/science/2018/03/amid-drug-price-increases-pfizer-ceo-gets-61-pay-raise-to-27-9-million/

22 B. Kenber, 'Pfizer "Exploited NHS Loophole" as Drug Price Rose 2,600%', *The Times*, 5 August 2021, https://www.thetimes.co.uk/article/pfizer-exploited-loophole-to-charge-nhs-higher-price-for-epilepsy-drug-b05j9vf9l

23 J. Ambrose and R. Davies, 'Pharma Firm Advanz Fined After Thyroid Drug Price Hike of 6,000%', *Guardian*, 29 July 2021, https://www.theguardian.com/business/2021/jul/29/pharma-firm-advanz-fined-after-thyroid-tablets-price-inflation-of-6000

24 'Mylan's EpiPen Pricing Scandal', Seven Pillars Institute, 14 September 2017, https://sevenpillarsinstitute.org/mylans-epipen-pricing-scandal/

25 'NICE Responds to Article in The Times', National Institute for Health and Care Excellence, 3 September 2013, https://www.nice.org.uk/news/article/nice-responds-to-article-in-the-times

26 J.A. DiMasi et al, 'Innovation in the Pharmaceutical Industry: New Estimates of R&D Costs', *Journal of Health Economics*, May 2016, http://www.sciencedirect.com/science/article/pii/S0167629616000291

27 'Financial Disclosure', Tufts Center for the Study of Drug Development, https://csdd.tufts.edu/financial-disclosure

28 V. Prasad, 'Research and Development Spending to Bring a Single Cancer Drug to Market and Revenues After Approval', *JAMA Internal Medicine*, November 2017, https://doi.org/10.1001/jamainternmed.2017.3601

29 E.G. Cleary et al, 'Contribution of NIH Funding to New Drug Approvals 2010–2016', *Proceedings of the National Academy of Sciences of the United States of America*, 6 March 2018, https://www.pnas.org/content/115/10/2329

30 'Pills and Profits: How Drug Companies Make a Killing Out of Public Research', Global Justice Now, https://www.globaljustice.org.uk/sites/default/files/files/news_article/pills-and-profits-report-web.pdf

31 M. Newman, 'Drug Companies Are Incentivised to Profit not to Improve Health, Says Report', *British Medical Journal*, 16 October 2018, https://www.bmj.com/content/363/bmj.k4351.full

32 Billy Kenber, *Sick Money*, Canongate, 2021

33 L.M. Schwartz and S. Woloshin, 'Medical Marketing in the United States, 1997–2016', *JAMA*, January 2019, https://jamanetwork.com/journals/jama/fullarticle/2720029

ENDNOTES

34 'Should Prescription Drugs Ads Be Reined In?', *New York Times*, 4 August 2009
35 'The United Nations Secretary-General's High-Level Panel on Access to Medicines Report', http://www.unsgaccessmeds.org/final-report/
36 S.G. Morgan, S. Vogler, A.K. Wagner, 'Payers' Experiences with Confidential Pharmaceutical Price Discounts: A Survey of Public and Statutory Health Systems in North America, Europe, and Australasia', *Health Policy*, 2017;121, pp. 354–62
37 'Essential Medicines and Health Products Information Portal', World Health Organization, http://apps.who.int/medicinedocs/documents/s19160en/s19160en.pdf
38 H. Burke, 'Who Are the Top 10 Pharmaceutical Companies in the World?', Proclinical, 6 July 2021, https://www.proclinical.com/blogs/2019-3/the-top-10-pharmaceutical-companies-in-the-world-2019#
39 'How Big Pharma made a Killing from the Coronavirus Pandemic', *The Times*, 2 October 2021
40 N. Pratley, 'Why AstraZeneca's Reward for Covid Vaccine is a Share Price Slump', *Guardian*, https://www.theguardian.com/business/nils-pratley-on-finance/2020/nov/23/why-astrazenecas-reward-for-covid-vaccine-is-a-share-price-slump
41 N. Burleigh, 'How The Covid-19 Vaccine Injected Billions Into Big Pharma – And Made Its Executives Very Rich', *Forbes*, 14 March 2021, https://www.forbes.com/sites/forbesdigitalcovers/2021/05/14/virus-book-excerpt-nina-burleigh-how-the-covid-19-vaccine-injected-billions-into-big-pharma-albert-bourla-moncef-slaoui/
42 K. Tay-Teo, A. Ilbawi and S.R. Hill, 'Comparison of Sales Income and Research and Development Costs for FDA-Approved Cancer Drugs Sold by Originator Drug Companies', *JAMA*, 4 January 2019, https://www.ncbi.nlm.nih.gov/pmc/articles/PMC6324319/
43 H.M. Kantarjian, T. Fojo, M. Mathisen and L.A. Zwelling, 'Cancer Drugs in the United States: Justum Pretium – the Just Price', *Journal of Clinical Oncology* 31, no. 28 (1 October 2013), pp. 3600–4.
44 C. David et al, 'Availability of Evidence of Benefits on Overall Survival and Quality of Life of Cancer Drugs Approved by European Medicines Agency: Retrospective Cohort Study of Drug Approvals 2009–13', *British Medical Journal*, 4 October 2017, https://www.bmj.com/content/359/bmj.j4530
45 V. Prasad, K. De Jesús and S. Mailankody, 'The High Price of Anticancer Drugs: Origins, Implications, Barriers, Solutions', *Nature Reviews Clinical Oncology*, 14 March 2017, https://doi.org/10.1038/nrclinonc.2017.31

46 Q. Chen et al, 'Economic Burden of Chronic Lymphocytic Leukemia in the Era of Oral Targeted Therapies in the United States', *Journal of Clinical Oncology*, November 2016, pp. 166–74

Chapter 5: Valuing a Life

1 L. Donnelly and P. Scott, 'Pill Nation: Half of Us Take at Least One Prescription Drug Daily', *Daily Telegraph*, 13 December 2007, https://www.telegraph.co.uk/news/2017/12/13/pill-nation-half-us-take-least-one-prescription-drug-daily/

2 'Nearly One in Two Americans Takes Prescription Drugs: Survey', Bloomberg, 7 May 2019, https://www.bloomberg.com/news/articles/2019-05-08/nearly-one-in-two-americans-takes-prescription-drugs-survey

3 'Prescription Cost Analysis – England, 2017 [PAS]', NHS Digital, 15 March 2018, https://digital.nhs.uk/data-and-information/publications/statistical/prescription-cost-analysis/prescription-cost-analysis-england-2017

4 K. Malik, 'The $2m Drug Reveals Medical Research as a Casino Culture', *Guardian*, 26 May 2019, https://www.theguardian.com/commentisfree/2019/may/26/gene-therapy-zolgensma-novartis

5 J. Chisholm, 'Doctors Will Have to Choose Who Gets Life-Saving Treatment. Here's How We'll Do It', *Guardian*, 1 April 2020, https://www.theguardian.com/commentisfree/2020/apr/01/doctors-choose-life-saving-treatment-ethical-rules

6 'COVID-19: Ethical Issues When Demand for Life-Saving Treatment is at Capacity', BMA, https://www.bma.org.uk/advice-and-support/covid-19/ethics/covid-19-ethical-issues

7 E. Batte, 'Dr Feelgood's Wilko Johnson Diagnosed With Terminal Cancer', Stereoboard.com, 9 January 2013, https://www.stereoboard.com/content/view/176753/9#ixzz2HUlhUnfy

8 M. McArdle, 'Opinion: The Truth about Medical Bankruptcies', *Washington Post*, 26 March 2018, 'https://www.washingtonpost.com/blogs/post-partisan/wp/2018/03/26/the-truth-about-medical-bankruptcies/

9 C. Dobkin et al, 'Myth and Measurement – The Case of Medical Bankruptcies', *The New England Journal of Medicine*, 22 March 2018, http://pnhp.org/blog/2018/03/22/the-myth-that-medical-bankruptcies-are-rare/

10 https://www.facebook.com/notes/sarah-palin/statement-on-the-current-health-care-debate/113851103434/

11 'Letters: Which Is Important – Money or Human Life?', *The Northern Echo*, 18 May 2018, https://www.thenorthernecho.co.uk/opinion/letters/16234582.letters-important---money-human-life/

ENDNOTES

12 S. Boseley, 'Patients Suffer When NHS Buys Expensive New Drugs, Says Report', *Guardian*, 19 February 2015, https://www.theguardian.com/society/2015/feb/19/nhs-buys-expensive-new-drugs-nice-york-karl-claxton-nice

13 https://www.nice.org.uk/Media/Default/About/what-we-do/Research-and-development/Social-Value-Judgements-principles-for-the-development-of-NICE-guidance.pdf

14 L.M. Sabik and R.K. Lie, 'Priority Setting in Health Care: Lessons from the Experiences of Eight Countries', *International Journal for Equity in Health*, January 2008, https://www.who.int/pmnch/topics/health_systems/200801_equityhealthj/en/

15 J. Geyman, 'Cost Effectiveness Analysis in US Healthcare – Long Overdue', *Huffington Post*, 17 June 2016

16 C. Kim, V. Prasad. 'Cancer Drugs Approved on the Basis of a Surrogate End Point and Subsequent Overall Survival: An Analysis of 5 Years of US Food and Drug Administration Approvals', *JAMA Internal Medicine*, 2015;359, pp. 1992–4

17 'Payers Report that ICER Analyses Increasingly Guide US Price Negotiations', ICON, 15 November 2019, https://www.iconplc.com/insights/blog/2019/11/15/payers-report-that-icer-analyses-increasingly-guide-us-price-negotiations/

18 M. Lokke, 'The New War on (Overpriced) Drugs', *Wired*, 10 June 2017, https://www.wired.com/story/fighting-high-drug-prices/

19 'How to Cut US Drug Prices: Experts Weigh In', *New York Times*, 10 December 2017, https://www.nytimes.com/2018/12/10/upshot/how-to-cut-drug-prices-experts-weigh-in.html

20 'In Cancer Care, Cost Matters', *New York Times*, 14 October 2012, https://www.canceradvocacy.org/wp-content/uploads/2013/10/Cost-of-Care-P-Back-L-Saltz-and-R-Wittes.pdf

Chapter 6: Better than Cure

1 R. Masters, E. Anwar, B. Collins et al, 'Return on Investment of Public Health Interventions: A Systematic Review', *Journal of Epidemiology and Community Health*, 2017;71, pp. 827–834.

2 'Prevention Is Better than Cure', Department of Health and Social Care, 5 November 2018, http://data.parliament.uk/DepositedPapers/Files/DEP2018-1087/Prevention_is_Better_than_Cure.pdf

3 D. Brady, 'Government Slammed for Public Health Grant Cuts', Public Finance, 21 December 2018, https://www.publicfinance.co.uk/news/2018/12/government-slammed-public-health-grant-cuts

4 'New Reductions to the Public Health Grant Will Heap More Pressure on Local Authorities', The Health Foundation, 20 December 2018, https://

ENDNOTES

www.health.org.uk/news-and-comment/news/new-reductions-to-the-public-health-grant-will-heap-more-pressure-on-local

5 L. Garrett, *Betrayal of Trust: The Collapse of Global Public Health*, Hachette Books, 2000
6 'Motorcycles', Traffic Safety Facts, February 2018, https://crashstats.nhtsa.dot.gov/Api/Public/ViewPublication/812492
7 'Helmet Use Among Motorcyclists Who Died in Crashes and Economic Cost Savings Associated with State Motorcycle Helmet Laws – United States, 2008–2010', Centers for Disease Control and Prevention, https://www.cdc.gov/mmwr/preview/mmwrhtml/mm6123a1.htm
8 N.E. McSwain Jr and A. Belles, 'Motorcycle Helmets – Medical Costs and the Law', *The Journal of Trauma*, October 1990, https://pubmed.ncbi.nlm.nih.gov/2120462/
9 A. Eltorai et al, 'Federally mandating motorcycle helmets in the United States', *BMC Public Health*, 9 March 2016, https://www.ncbi.nlm.nih.gov/pmc/articles/PMC4784405/
10 F.P. Rivara, B.G. Dicker, A.B. Bergman, R. Dacey, C. Herman, 'The Public Cost of Motorcycle Trauma', *JAMA*, 8 July 1988, https://pubmed.ncbi.nlm.nih.gov/3290518/
11 J.C. Hundley, P.D. Kilgo, P.R. Miller, M.C. Chang, R.A. Hensberry, J.W. Meredith et al, 'Non-Helmeted Motorcyclists: A Burden to Society?', *The Journal of Trauma*, November 2004, https://journals.lww.com/jtrauma/Abstract/2004/11000/Non_Helmeted_Motorcyclists__A_Burden_to_Society__A.4.aspx
12 O. Milman, 'Mandatory Bike Helmet Laws Do More Harm Than Good, Senate Hears', *Guardian*, 12 August 2015, https://www.theguardian.com/lifeandstyle/2015/aug/12/mandatory-bike-helmet-laws-do-more-harm-than-good-senate-hears
13 J. Hughes, 'Mandatory Helmet Laws Across The US', 6 April 2019, https://www.rideapart.com/articles/337084/mandatory-helmet-laws-across-us/
14 A.H. Mokdad, J.S. Marks, D.F. Stroup, J.L. Gerberding, 'Actual Causes of Death in the United States', *Journal of the American Medical Association*, 2004;291(10), pp. 1238–45.
15 'At Work', a quarterly publication of the Institute for Work and Health, Spring 2015, https://www.iwh.on.ca/sites/iwh/files/iwh/at-work/at_work_80_0.pdf
16 https://www.nice.org.uk/Media/Default/About/what-we-do/NICE-International/projects/67th-WHA-full-speech-by-David-Haslam.pdf
17 'The Primary Health Care Performance Initiative', PHCPI, https://improvingphc.org/about-phcpi

ENDNOTES

18 'For an Inclusive, Evidence-Based and Sustainable G7 Action in Global Health', 17 May 2019, https://www.gouvernement.fr/en/for-an-inclusive-evidence-based-and-sustainable-g7-action-in-global-health

19 J. Campbell, 'Provision of Primary Care in Different Countries', *British Medical Journal*, 16 June 2007, https://www.ncbi.nlm.nih.gov/pmc/articles/PMC1892491/

20 https://www.who.int/healthinfo/universal_health_coverage/report/2019/en/

21 J. Silberner, 'Increase Investment in Primary Healthcare by 1% of GDP, Says WHO', *British Medical Journal*, 23 September 2019, https://www.bmj.com/content/366/bmj.l5664.full

22 B. Starfield, S. Leiyu and J. Macinko, 'Contribution of Primary Care to Health Systems and Health', *The Millbank Quarterly*, September 2005, https://www.ncbi.nlm.nih.gov/pmc/articles/PMC2690145/

23 M. Lakhani (ed), 'The Effectiveness of Primary Healthcare', in *A Celebration of General Practice*, Radcliffe Medical Press, 2003

24 D. Haslam, '"Schools and Hospitals" for "Education and Health"', *British Medical Journal*, 1 February 2003, https://doi.org/10.1136/bmj.326.7383.234

25 https://www.longtermplan.nhs.uk

26 S. Basu, S.A. Berkowitz, R.L. Phillips et al, 'Association of Primary Care Physician Supply With Population Mortality in the United States, 2005–2015', *JAMA Internal Medicine*, 18 February 2019, https://jamanetwork.com/journals/jamainternalmedicine/fullarticle/2724393

27 L. Rapaport, 'Supply of Primary Care Doctors Linked with Mortality Rates', Reuters, 18 February 2019, https://uk.reuters.com/article/us-health-primary-care/supply-of-primary-care-doctors-linked-with-mortality-rates-idUKKCN1Q71NC

28 'The NHS Workforce in Numbers', Nuffield Trust, 8 May 2019, https://www.nuffieldtrust.org.uk/resource/the-nhs-workforce-in-numbers

29 B. Jarman, S. Gault, B. Alves, A. Hider, S. Dolan, A. Cook, B. Hurwitz, L. Iezzoni, 'Explaining Differences in English Hospital Death Rates Using Routinely Collected Data', *British Medical Journal*, 1999, 318, pp. 1515–20

30 M. Marmot et al, 'Fair Society Healthy Lives (The Marmot Review)', Institute of Health Equity, February 2010, http://www.instituteofhealthequity.org/resources-reports/fair-society-healthy-lives-the-marmot-review

31 Ibid

32 G.K. Singh et al, 'Social Determinants of Health in the United States: Addressing Major Health Inequality Trends for the Nation, 1935–2016', *The International Journal of Maternal and Child Health and AIDS*, 2017, https://www.ncbi.nlm.nih.gov/pmc/articles/PMC5777389/

ENDNOTES

33 'Social Determinants of Health', Australian Institute of Health and Welfare, https://www.aihw.gov.au/getmedia/746ded57-183a-40e9-8bdb-828e21203175/aihw-aus-221-chapter-4-2.pdf.aspx

34 'Social Determinants of Health and Health Inequalities', Government of Canada, https://www.canada.ca/en/public-health/services/health-promotion/population-health/what-determines-health.html

Chapter 7: Overtreatment and Overdiagnosis

1 J.M.G. Wilson and G. Jungner, 'Principles and Practice of Screening for disease', *WHO Chronicle*, 1968

2 '2017 Guideline for the Prevention, Detection, Evaluation, and Management of High Blood Pressure in Adults', American College of Cardiology, https://www.acc.org/-/media/Non-Clinical/Files-PDFs-Excel-MS-Word-etc/Guidelines/2017/Guidelines_Made_Simple_2017_HBP.pdf

3 R. Khera et al, 'Impact of 2017 ACC/AHA Guidelines on Prevalence of Hypertension and Eligibility for Antihypertensive Treatment in United States and China: Nationally Representative Cross Sectional Study', *British Medical Journal*, 11 July 2018, https://www.bmj.com/content/362/bmj.k2357

4 J.M. Wright and V.M. Musini, 'First-Line Drugs for Hypertension', *Cochrane Database of Systematic Reviews*, 2009;(3):CD001841

5 'Suicides in the UK: 2018 Registrations', Office for National Statistics, 3 September 2019, https://www.ons.gov.uk/peoplepopulationandcommunity/birthsdeathsandmarriages/deaths/bulletins/suicidesintheunitedkingdom/2018registrations

6 'Medicalising Unhappiness: New Classification of Depression Risks More Patients Being Put on Drug Treatment from Which They Will not Benefit', *British Medical Journal*, 9 December 2013

7 https://www.diabetes.co.uk/pre-diabetes.html

8 A.G Mainous III, R.J. Tanner, R. Baker, C.E. Zayas, C.A Harle, 'Prevalence of Prediabetes in England from 2003 to 2011: Population-Based, Cross-Sectional Study', *BMJ Open*, https://bmjopen.bmj.com/content/4/6/e005002

9 J. Yudkin and V. Montori, 'The Epidemic of Pre-Diabetes: The Medicine and the Politics', *British Medical Journal*, 16 July 2014, https://www.ncbi.nlm.nih.gov/pmc/articles/PMC4707710/

10 https://www.agreetrust.org

11 https://www.england.nhs.uk/shared-decision-making/

12 'Taking a Statin to Reduce the Risk of Coronary Heart Disease and Stroke', National Institute for Health and Care Excellence, November 2014, https://www.nice.org.uk/guidance/cg181/resources/patient-decision-aid-pdf-243780159

13 J. Treadwell et al, 'GPs' Understanding of the Benefits and Harms of Treatments for Long-Term Conditions: An Online Survey', *BJSP Open*, April 2020, https://doi.org/10.3399/bjgpopen20X101016
14 T.C. Hoffmann, C. Del Mar, 'Patients' Expectations of the Benefits and Harms of Treatments, Screening, and Tests: A Systematic Review', *JAMA Internal Medicine*, 2015;175(2):274–286, https://pubmed.ncbi.nlm.nih.gov/25531451/
15 M. Blastland, 'The Dark Side of Early Diagnosis', *Prospect*, 22 August 2018, https://www.prospectmagazine.co.uk/magazine/early-diagnosis-cancer-screening-women-risk
16 http://understandinguncertainty.org/visualisation-information-nhs-breast-cancer-screening-leaflet
17 M. Blastland, 'The Dark Side of Early Diagnosis', *Prospect*, 22 August 2018
18 P. Glasziou et al, 'Estimating the Magnitude of Cancer Overdiagnosis in Australia', *MJA*, 6 April 2020, https://www.mja.com.au/journal/2020/212/4/estimating-magnitude-cancer-overdiagnosis-australia
19 J. Brodersen et al, 'Overdiagnosis: What it Is and What it Isn't', *BMJ Evidence-Based Medicine*, https://ebm.bmj.com/content/23/1/1
20 J. Brodersen, L.M. Schwartz, S. Woloshin, 'Overdiagnosis: How Cancer Screening Can Turn Indolent Pathology into Illness', *APMIS*, 2014;122: 683–9, doi:10.1111/apm.12278
21 S. Park, C.M. Oh, H. Cho et al, 'Association Between Screening and the Thyroid Cancer "Epidemic" in South Korea: Evidence from a Nationwide Study', *British Medical Journal*, 2016;355:i5745, doi:10.1136/bmj.i5745
22 'Patients' Preferences Matter: Stop the Silent Misdiagnosis', The King's Fund, 29 May 2012, https://www.kingsfund.org.uk/publications/patients-preferences-matter
23 L. Payer, *Disease-Mongers: How Doctors, Drug Companies and Insurers Are Making You Feel Sick*, Wiley, 1992
24 http://www.europarl.europa.eu/RegData/etudes/note/join/2012/492462/IPOL-ENVI_NT(2012)492462_EN.pdf
25 'Widespread Debate Needed on "Disease Mongering" and Overdiagnosis of Patients, Says RCGP in Response to BMJ Evidence-Based Medicine Paper on Definitions of Disease', Royal College of GPs, 8 April 2019, https://www.rcgp.org.uk/about-us/news/2019/april/widespread-debate-needed-on-disease-mongering-and-overdiagnosis-of-patients-says-rcgp.aspx
26 'Unnecessary Care in Canada: Infographic', CIHI, https://www.cihi.ca/en/unnecessary-care-in-canada-infographic
27 T. Pathirana et al, '8 Drivers and Potential Solutions for Overdiagnosis: Perspectives from the Low and Middle Income Countries', *BMJ Evidence-Based Medicine*, https://ebm.bmj.com/content/24/Suppl_2/A6.2

ENDNOTES

28. J. Andriote, 'Legal Drug-Pushing: How Disease Mongers Keep Us All Doped Up', *The Atlantic*, 3 April 2012, https://www.theatlantic.com/health/archive/2012/04/legal-drug-pushing-how-disease-mongers-keep-us-all-doped-up/255247/
29. R. Moynihan, I. Heath, D. Henry, 'Selling Sickness: The Pharmaceutical Industry and Disease Mongering', *British Medical Journal*, 2002;324(7342):886–891

Chapter 8: Hearts and Minds

1. 'Mental Health Funding Squeeze has Lengthened Waiting Times, Say NHS Finance Leads', The King's Fund, 21 December 2018, https://www.kingsfund.org.uk/press/press-releases/mental-health-funding-squeeze-has-lengthened-waiting-times-say-nhs-finance
2. 'Tired Of The Wait: ER Doctors Make the Case for Mental Health Reform', NAMI, 25 October 2016, https://www.nami.org/About-NAMI/NAMI-News/2016/Tired-of-the-Wait
3. E. Anderssen, 'How to Fix Canada's Mental Health System', *The Globe and Mail*, 1 June 2015, https://beta.theglobeandmail.com/news/national/how-to-fix-canadas-mental-health-system/article24733006
4. A. Brown, 'Death Rate for People Seeking Mental Health Treatment Double the Australian Rate', *Canberra Times*, 16 September 2017, https://www.canberratimes.com.au/story/6028273/death-rate-for-people-seeking-mental-health-treatment-double-the-australian-rate/
5. P. Wang et al, 'Delay and Failure in Treatment Seeking After First Onset of Mental Disorders in the World Health Organization's World Mental Health Survey Initiative', *World Psychiatry*, October 2007, https://www.ncbi.nlm.nih.gov/pmc/articles/PMC2174579/
6. N. Triggle, 'Hidden Waits "Leave Mental Health Patients in Limbo"', BBC News, 5 December 2019, https://www.bbc.co.uk/news/health-50658007
7. 'Daily Insight: Hundreds of Children Languish on Waiting Lists', *HSJ*, 31 August 2018, https://www.hsj.co.uk/daily-insight/daily-insight-hundreds-of-children-languish-on-waiting-lists/7023252.article
8. E. Bullmore, 'From Depression to Dementia, Inflammation Is Medicine's New Frontier', *Guardian*, 19 January 2020, https://www.theguardian.com/commentisfree/2020/jan/19/inflammation-depression-mind-body
9. J. McNamara, M. Molot, J. Stremple et al, 'Coronary Artery Disease in Combat Casualties in Vietnam', *JAMA*, 1971;216(7):1185–1187, https://jamanetwork.com/journals/jama/article-abstract/336112
10. 'Coronary Heart Disease', Health Knowledge, https://www.healthknowledge.org.uk/public-health-textbook/disease-causation-diagnostic/2b-epidemiology-diseases-phs/chronic-diseases/coronary-heart-disease

ENDNOTES

11 C. Fryar, T. Chen, X. Li, 'Prevalence of Uncontrolled Risk Factors for Cardiovascular Disease: United States, 1999–2010', *NCHS Data Brief*, August 2012, https://www.cdc.gov/nchs/data/databriefs/db103.pdf

12 J. Wang et al, 'Prevalence of Depression and Depressive Symptoms Among Outpatients: A Systematic Review and Meta-Analysis', *Mental Health Research*, http://dx.doi.org/10.1136/bmjopen-2017-017173

13 'Global, Regional and National Incidence, Prevalence and Years Lived with Disability for 310 Diseases and Injuries, 1990–2015: A Systematic Analysis for the Global Burden of Disease Study 2015', *The Lancet*, 2016;388:1545–602, doi:10.1016/S0140-6736(16)31678-6

14 'The World Health Report 2002: Reducing Risks, Promoting Healthy Life', World Health Organization, 2002

15 D.C. Kuo, M. Tran, A.A Shah et al, 'Depression and the Suicidal Patient', *Emergency Medicine Clinics of North America*, 2015;33:765–78, doi:10.1016/j.emc.2015.07.005

16 https://www.nras.org.uk/invisible-disease-rheumatoid-arthritis-and-chronic-fatigue-report

17 B.A. Kitchener, A.F. Jorm, C.M Kelly, 'Mental Health First Aid International Manual', Mental Health First Aid International, 2015

Chapter 9: Age and Ageing

1 D. Levitin, *The Changing Mind*, Penguin, 2020
2 https://www.un.org/en/sections/issues-depth/ageing/
3 'Overview of the UK population: August 2019', Office for National Statistics, 23 August 2019, https://www.ons.gov.uk/peoplepopulationandcommunity/populationandmigration/populationestimates/articles/overviewoftheukpopulation/august2019#main-points
4 B. Bryson, *The Body*, Doubleday, 2019
5 D. Lieberman, *The Story of the Human Body: Evolution, Health & Disease*, Penguin, 2014
6 D. Levitin, *The Changing Mind*, Penguin, 2020
7 *The World Health Report: Report of the Director-General*, World Health Organization, Geneva, Switzerland, 1997
8 V. Raleigh, 'What Is Happening to Life Expectancy in England?', The King's Fund, 6 December 2021, https://www.kingsfund.org.uk/publications/whats-happening-life-expectancy-uk
9 E. Wigger, 'The Whitehall Study', The Center for Social Epidemiology, https://unhealthywork.org/classic-studies/the-whitehall-study/
10 https://www.mhlw.go.jp/english/wp/wp-hw2/part2/p2c1s3.pd

ENDNOTES

11 'Investigative Research Report on Innovation Using AI/IoT in the Health, Healthcare, and Nursing Care Fields', Institute for International Socio-Economic Studies

12 S. Watanabe, 'Longevity and Elderly Care: Lessons from Japan', *Global Health Journal*, December 2018, https://www.sciencedirect.com/science/article/pii/S2414644719301770#bib9

13 'OECD Reviews of Public Health: Japan', Organization for Economic Co-operation and Development, https://www.oecd.org/health/health-systems/OECD-Reviews-of-Public-Health-Japan-Assessment-and-recommendations.pdf

14 'Multiple Illnesses and End-of-Life Care Drive High Healthcare Costs in Old Age', National Institute for Health Research, 24 October 2017, https://discover.dc.nihr.ac.uk/content/signal-000496/multiple-illnesses-and-end of life-care-drive-high-healthcare-costs-in-old-age

15 'Compassionate Community Project', *Resurgence & Ecologist*, March 2018

16 Health Connections Mendip, https://healthconnectionsmendip.org

17 L. Entis, 'Scientists Are Working on a Pill for Loneliness', *Guardian*, 26 January 2019, https://www.theguardian.com/us-news/2019/jan/26/pill-for-loneliness-psychology-science-medicine

18 S. Jain, 'A Treatment for Loneliness', *Harvard Medicine*, https://hms.harvard.edu/magazine/imaging/treatment-loneliness

19 D. Haslam, 'Who Cares? The James Mackenzie Lecture 2006', *British Journal of General Practice*, 2007;57 (545): 987–993, https://bjgp.org/content/57/545/987

20 D. Buck and L. Ewbank, 'What Is Social Prescribing?', The King's Fund, 4 November 2020, https://www.kingsfund.org.uk/publications/social-prescribing

21 L. Donnelly, 'Doctors Are Replacing the Roles that Used to Be Done by Priests and Barmaids, Says the NHS's Head of Social Prescribing', *Daily Telegraph*, 20 January 2020, https://www.telegraph.co.uk/news/2020/01/20/doctors-replacing-roles-used-done-priests-barmaids-says-nhss/

22 M.J. Polley, et al, 'Making Sense of Social Prescribing', https://westminsterresearch.westminster.ac.uk/item/q1v77/making-sense-of-social-prescribing

23 R. Mead, 'What Britain's "Minister of Loneliness" Says About Brexit and the Legacy of Jo Cox', *New Yorker*, 26 January 2018, https://www.newyorker.com/culture/cultural-comment/britain-minister-of-loneliness-brexit-jo-cox

24 S. McBain, 'How Loneliness Became an Epidemic', *New Statesman*, 2 January 2020

25 R. Dantzer, J.C. O'Connor, G.G. Freund, R.W. Johnson, K.W. Kelley, 'From Inflammation to Sickness and Depression: When the Immune System

Subjugates the Brain', *National Review of Neuroscience*, 2008;9(1):46–56, doi:10.1038/nrn2297

26 J. Holt-Lunstad, 'Social Relationships and Mortality Risk: A Meta-analytic Review', *PLOS Medicine*, 27 July 2010, https://journals.plos.org/plosmedicine/article?id=10.1371/journal.pmed.1000316

27 B. Ehrenreich, *Natural Causes: Life, Death and the Illusion of Control*, London, Granta Books, 2019

Chapter 10: And in the End …

1 O. Jones, 'End-of-Life Care Is Vital. Why Is it so Neglected?', *Guardian*, 31 January 2020, https://www.theguardian.com/commentisfree/2020/jan/31/end of life-care-britain-palliative-charity-public

2 'End of Life Care Strategy: Fourth Annual Report', Department of Health, https://www.gov.uk/government/uploads/system/uploads/attachment_data/file/136486/End of life-Care-Strategy-Fourth-Annual-report-web-version-v2.pdf

3 'End of Life Care Strategy: Promoting High-Quality Care for All Adults at the End of Life', Department of Health

4 'Ambitions for Palliative and End of Life Care: A National Framework for Local Action 2021–2026', National Palliative and End of Life Care Partnership, May 2021, https://www.sueryder.org/sites/default/files/2021-06/Ambitions-for-Palliative-and-End-of-Life-Care-2nd-Edition.pdf

5 https://www.gov.uk/government/publications/end of life-care-profiles-february-2018-update/statistical-commentary-end of life-care-profiles-february-2018-update

6 https://www.hospiceuk.org/about-hospice-care/media-centre/facts-and-figures

7 'Annual Review of Public Health', Volume 35, 2014, pp. 459–75

8 A. Dose et al, 'Dying in the Hospital: Perspectives of family members', *Journal of Palliative Care*, 2015;31(1):13–20, https://www.ncbi.nlm.nih.gov/pubmed/26399086

9 A. Gawande, *Being Mortal*, Profile Books, 2014

10 https://richardswsmith.wordpress.com/2018/09/25/why-do-doctors-abandon-the-dying/

11 D. Oliver, 'Progressive Dwindling, Frailty and Realistic Expectations', *British Medical Journal*, 2017;358:j3954

12 E. Hutt, A Da Silva, E. Bogart, S. Le Lay-Doimande, D. Pannier, S. Delaine-Clisant, M. Le Deley, A. Adenis, 'Impact of Early Palliative Care on Overall Survival of Patients with Metastatic Upper Gastrointestinal Cancers Treated with First-Line Chemotherapy: A Randomised Phase III Trial', *British*

ENDNOTES

      Medical Journal, 1 May 2019, https://bmjopen.bmj.com/content/8/1/e015904

13. A. Wright et al, 'Associations Between End-of-Life Discussions, Patient Mental Health, Medical Care Near Death and Caregiver Bereavement Adjustment', *JAMA*, 8 October 2008, https://www.ncbi.nlm.nih.gov/pmc/articles/PMC2853806/
14. https://www.nmc.org.uk/news/news-and-updates/reflections-on-recent-cpr-fitness-to-practise-case/
15. D. Oliver, 'Keeping Care Home Residents out of Hospital', *British Medical Journal*, 2016;358 pmid:26813928
16. https://twitter.com/SDenegri/status/1196001876858343424
17. 'Do Cancer Drugs Improve Survival or Quality of Life?', *British Medical Journal*, 2017;359:j4528
18. C. Davis et al, 'Availability of Evidence of Benefits on Overall Survival and Quality of Life of Cancer Drugs Approved by European Medicines Agency: Retrospective Cohort Study of Drug Approvals 2009–13', *British Medical Journal*, 4 October 2017, https://www.bmj.com/content/359/bmj.j4530
19. G, Sanderson, 'Excess Deaths at Home Not Driven By Covid', *The Times*, https://www.thetimes.co.uk/article/excess-deaths-at-home-not-driven-by-covid-ons-says-5tsrhx0lw

Chapter 11: Care in the Future

1. F. Collins, 'Has the Revolution Arrived?', *Nature*, 2010;464(7289):674–675, doi:10.1038/464674a
2. 'The Future of Employment: How Susceptible Are Jobs to Computerisation?', Oxford Martin School, University of Oxford, https://www.oxfordmartin.ox.ac.uk/publications/the-future-of-employment/
3. M. Britnell, *Human: Solving the Global Workforce Crisis in Healthcare*, Oxford University Press, 2019
4. doi: 10.1136/bmjopen-2019-032412
5. 'All GP Consultations Should Be Remote by Default, Says Matt Hancock', *Guardian*, 30 July 2020
6. M. Marshall, RCGP Weekly Digest, 26 June 2020
7. H. Vogt, S. Green, C. Thorn Ekstrøm, J. Broderson, 'How Precision Medicine and Screening with Big Data Could Increase Overdiagnosis', *British Medical Journal*, 13 September 2019, https://doi.org/10.1136/bmj.l5270
8. D. Ariely, Facebook, https://www.facebook.com/dan.ariely/posts/904383595868

ENDNOTES

9 A. Hosny, C. Parmar, J. Quackenbush, L. Schwartz and H. Aerts, 'Artificial Intelligence in Radiology', *Nature Reviews Cancer*, August 2018, https://www.ncbi.nlm.nih.gov/pmc/articles/PMC6268174/

10 P. Mistry, 'Artificial Intelligence in Primary Care', *British Journal of General Practice*, September 2019, pp. 422–3

11 'Robots to Be Used in UK Care Homes to Help Reduce Loneliness', *Guardian*, 7 September 2020, https://www.theguardian.com/society/2020/sep/07/robots-used-uk-care-homes-help-reduce-loneliness

12 D. Keltner, 'Hands On Research: The Science of Touch', *Greater Good Magazine*, 29 September 2010, https://greatergood.berkeley.edu/article/item/hands_on_research

13 S. Davies, 'Generation Genome', *Annual Report of the Chief Medical Officer 2016*, https://assets.publishing.service.gov.uk/government/uploads/system/uploads/attachment_data/file/631043/CMO_annual_report_generation_genome.pdf

14 *The New England Journal of Medicine*, 2021;385:1868–1880, doi: 10.1056/NEJMoa2035790

15 https://grail.com

16 'Direct-to-Consumer Genetic Testing', *British Medical Journal*, 16 October 2019, https://doi.org/10.1136/bmj.l5688

17 'Seeing the Future? How Genetic Testing Will Impact Life Insurance', Swiss Re Institute, https://www.swissre.com/dam/jcr:2bccf1e2-eaa5-4ca2-a416-f6dedcebe9dc/Genetics_Seeing_the_future.pdf

18 D. Dickenson, '*Me* medicine could undermine public health measures', *New Scientist*, 11 September 2013, https://www.newscientist.com/article/mg21929340-200-me-medicine-could-undermine-public-health-measures/#.UjhfPGSY5tI

19 R. Maziarz, 'CAR T-Cell Therapy Total Cost Can Exceed $1.5 million per Treatment', *Healio News*, 29 May 2019, https://www.healio.com/hematology-oncology/cell-therapy/news/online/%7B124396e7-1b60-4cff-a404-0a2baeaf1413%7D/car-t-cell-therapy-total-cost-can-exceed-15-million-per-treatment

Chapter 12: A Way Forward

1 G. Privitera, 'Italian doctors on coronavirus frontline face tough calls on whom to save', *Politico*, 9 March 2020, https://www.politico.eu/article/coronavirus-italy-doctors-tough-calls-survival/

2 J. Shaw, 'A Reformation for Our Times', *British Medical Journal*, 2009;338:b1080

3 Kar P, *British Medical Journal*, 2021;373:n989

ENDNOTES

4 D. Wanless, 'Securing our Future Health: Taking a Long-Term View', April 2002, https://www.yearofcare.co.uk/sites/default/files/images/Wanless.pdf
5 'Doctors to Prescribe Bike Rides to Tackle UK Obesity Crisis', *Guardian*, 26 July 2020, https://www.theguardian.com/politics/2020/jul/26/doctors-to-prescribe-bike-rides-to-tackle-uk-obesity-crisis-amid-coronavirus-risk
6 'The Frome Model', Compassionate Communities UK, https://www.compassionate-communitiesuk.co.uk/projects
7 J. Abel, H. Kingston, A. Scally, J. Hartnoll, G. Hannam, A, Thomson-Moore and A. Kellehear, 'Reducing Emergency Hospital Admissions: A Population Health Complex Intervention of an Enhanced Model of Primary Care and Compassionate Communities', *British Journal of General Practice*, 2018, https://doi.org/10.3399/bjgp18X699437
8 D. Callahan and S. Nuland, 'The Quagmire: How American medicine is destroying itself', *The New Republic*, 19 May 2011, https://newrepublic.com/article/88631/american-medicine-health-care-costs
9 A. Gawande, 'The Cost Conundrum', *New Yorker*, 1 June 2009
10 doi: 10.1186/s12916-016-0747-7
11 'NICE "Do Not Do" Recommendations', Nottingham Healthcare NHS Trust, https://www.nice.org.uk/media/default/sharedlearning/716_716donotdobookletfinal.pdf
12 'The 5 Most-viewed NICE "Do Not Do" Recommendations', National Institute for Health and Care Excellence, 1 December 2014, https://www.nice.org.uk/news/blog/the-5-most-viewed-nice-do-not-do-recommendations
13 'Cut NHS Waste Through NICE's "Do Not Do" Database', National Institute for Health and Care Excellence, 6 November 2014, https://www.nice.org.uk/news/article/cut-nhs-waste-through-nice-s--do-not-do--database
14 W. Shrank, T. Rogstad and N. Parekh, 'Waste in the US Health Care System: Estimated Costs and Potential for Savings', *JAMA*, 7 October 2019, https://jamanetwork.com/journals/jama/article-abstract/2752664
15 'Tackling Wasteful Spending on Health', Organization for Economic Cooperation and Development, https://www.oecd.org/els/health-systems/Tackling-Wasteful-Spending-on-Health-Highlights-revised.pdf
16 'Operational Productivity and Performance in English NHS Acute Hospitals: Unwarranted Variations', February 2016, https://assets.publishing.service.gov.uk/government/uploads/system/uploads/attachment_data/file/499229/Operational_productivity_A.pdf
17 Getting It Right First Time, https://gettingitrightfirsttime.co.uk/what-we-do/
18 J. Álvarez, R. Flores, J. Álvarez Grau, J. Matarranz, 'Process Reengineering and Patient-Centered Approach Strengthen Efficiency in Specialized Care', *The American Journal of Managed Care*, February 2019, Volume 25, Issue 2

ENDNOTES

19 P. Taylor, 'US Start-up EQRx Promises Approach that Will Slash Drug Prices', *PM Live*, 13 January 2020, http://www.pmlive.com/pharma_news/us_start-up_eqrx_promises_approach_that_will_slash_drug_prices_1322138

20 A. Tatsioni, N. Bonitsis, J. Ionannidis, 'Persistence of Contradicted Claims in the Literature', *JAMA*, 2007;298(21):2517–2526, https://jamanetwork.com/journals/jama/fullarticle/209653

21 P. Ubel, A. Angott and B. Zikmund-Fischer, 'Physicians Recommend Different Treatments for Patients Than They Would Choose for Themselves', *Archives of Internal Medicine*, 5 November 2013, https://www.ncbi.nlm.nih.gov/pmc/articles/PMC3817828/

22 'Patients' Preferences Matter: Stop the Silent Misdiagnosis', The King's Fund, 29 May 2012, https://www.kingsfund.org.uk/publications/patients-preferences-matter

23 N. Herodotou, *The Times*, 27 October 2021

24 N. Crisp, 'What Would a Sustainable Health and Care System Look Like?', *British Medical Journal*, 2017;358

25 V. Montori, 'Why We Revolt', patientrevolution.org

26 'General Practice in the Years Ahead', *British Journal of General Practice*, January 2021

27 'Martin Marshall Addresses RCGP Fresh Approach Online Conference', Royal College of General Practitioners, 11 February 2021, https://www.rcgp.org.uk/about-us/news/2021/february/martin-marshall-addresses-rcgp-fresh-approach-online-conference.aspx

28 S. MacLeod, 'The Future Doctor – Touching Hearts and Minds', https://doi.org/10.3399/bjgp21X71764

29 'What Is Personalised Care?', NHS England, https://www.england.nhs.uk/personalisedcare/what-is-personalised-care/

Index

Abel, Julian, 199
Academy of Medical Royal Colleges, 246
Actimmune (drug), 111
adalimumab (drug), 102
Advanz (pharmaceutical company), 95
age and ageing, 54–8, 85, 91, 190–205
   depression, 203–4
   disease span, 193–4
   'healthy life expectancy', 194–8
   loneliness, 199–203
   'social prescribing', 201–2
   see also end-of-life care; life expectancy
All Party Parliamentary Group on Longevity, 11
Allbutt, Clifford, 49
Alma-Ata, Kazakhstan, 60, 146
Alzheimer's disease, 242
American College of Emergency Physicians, 181
American Heart Association, 51
American Institute of Cancer Research, 33
anaemia, 34–5, 239
angioplasty, 53–4, 66
Appleby, John, 28
Appraisal of Guidelines for Research and Evaluation (AGREE), 165
Aranda, Sanchia, 172
Archives of Internal Medicine, 254
Ariely, Dan, 229

Arrow, Kenneth, 31–2
arthroscopy, 87
artificial intelligence (AI), 223, 229–30
aspirin, 110, 133
AstraZeneca (pharmaceutical company), 95, 106
Atlantic magazine, 177
austerity politics (UK), 4, 10, 25, 40
Australia, 59, 66, 75, 128–9, 138, 152–3, 171–2, 181
autism, 140
automation, 223–4
'availability heuristics', 88
Avastin (drug), 232
AveXis (pharmaceutical company), 111
Avorn, Jerry, 102

Bach, Peter, 132
Bagley, Nicholas, 132
Basu, Sanjay, 148
Being Mortal (Gawande), 209
Beloved Physician, The, 48, 50
Betrayal of Trust (Garrett), 136
Bevan, Aneurin, 58, 63, 73
Beveridge Report (1942), 28
BGI Group, 233
'big data' screening, 227–9
'Big Pharma', 94
von Bismarck, Otto, 70
Blackburn, Elizabeth, 54
Blair, Tony, 217

INDEX

Borisy, Alexis, 250
Brazil, 12, 81
Brexit, 202
British Medical Association (BMA), 116–17
British Medical Journal, 99, 108, 147, 160, 162–3, 177–8, 187, 211, 215, 228
Britnell, Mark, 223
Brown, Gordon, 242
Bryson, Bill, 193
Bullmore, Edward, 183
Bush, Barbara, 210

Callahan, Daniel, 246
Cameron, David, 25
Canada, 56, 59, 75, 153, 177, 181, 251, 253
cancer, 15, 27, 30–31, 33, 46–7, 52–3, 180–81, 242
  anti-cancer drugs, 107–9, 114, 127–8, 132, 215–16
  breast cancer screening, 168–70
  chimeric antigen receptor T-cell therapy, 108, 236–7
  genetic testing, 234–6
  palliative care, 211–12
  prostate cancer screening, 172–3
  thyroid cancer, 174
Cancer Drugs Fund (CDF), 119, 127, 183
Cancer Research UK, 30
  Early Detection Centre, 169
cardiopulmonary resuscitation, 115–16
cardiovascular disease, 43, 45–7, 50–54, 185–6
  coronary heart disease (CHD), 50–51, 185–6
  heart attacks, 43–4, 50, 53
  strokes, 43, 45
Castro, Fidel, 77

Centre for Ageing Better, 198–9
cervical smear tests, 157
Chan, Margaret, 68
Changing Mind, The (Levitin), 193
Chantler, Cyril, 47
Charles, Prince of Wales, 9
Chenodal (drug), 111
chimeric antigen receptor T-cell therapy, 108, 236–7
China, 75–6, 160, 163
cholera, 3, 48, 135
'Choosing Wisely' campaign, 252–4
Churchill, Winston, 49
'churnalism', 177–8
Cicero, 2, 191
Cinryze (drug), 111
citizens' assembly, 251
Claxton, Karl, 124
Clinton, Bill, 217
community action, 199, 201, 252–3
community care, 242, 244–5
Compassionate Communities project, 244–5
computerized medical records, 221–2
continuity of care, 258–9
'Coping with Cancer' project (US), 212
coronary heart disease, *see* cardiovascular disease
coronavirus, *see* Covid-19 pandemic
cost-effectiveness analysis (CEA), 119–30
Cota, Carrie, 29
Covid-19 pandemic, 1–6, 9–11, 21, 115, 218, 220
  costs of, 2, 5–6, 19
  impact on healthcare systems, 36–7, 238–9
  impact on life expectancy, 39–41
  lockdown, 4
  long Covid, 6
  Nightingale hospitals, 9–10, 13

INDEX

social distancing, 231
social inequality and, 11–12, 151
vaccines, 13, 19, 106–7, 252
crash helmets, 137–8
Crisp, Nigel, 257
Cronkite, Walter, 79
Crossman, Richard, 58
Cuba, 77–8
Cuomo, Andrew, 2
cytokines, 203–4

Daily Mail, 190
Daily Telegraph, 23
Daraprim (drug), 111
Davies, Sally, 232
De Senectute (Cicero), 191
'death panels', 113, 118–19
death, *see* end-of-life care
'defensive medicine', 88
dementia, 27, 47, 52
Denmark, 70
depression, *see* mental health
deprivation, *see* social inequality
diabetes, 29, 162–3, 242
Diabetes UK, 162–3
diagnosis 34–5, 157, 162, 168–70, 178–9, 233
  overdiagnosis, 155, 158–64, 170, 172–3, 175–7, 228–9
  'preference misdiagnosis', 174, 254–5
diarrhoea, 46
digital consulting, 225–7
Dillon, Andrew, 97–8
Dinutuximab Beta (drug), 119–20
diphtheria, 3, 48
'disease mongering', 175–7
doctors, 16–17, 150, 260
  digital consulting, 225–7
  GPs (General Practitioners), 3, 16–17, 48–50, 61–2, 146, 148–50, 221–2, 260

Quality and Outcomes Framework (QOF), 221–2
Donne, John, 252
Down's syndrome, 42
Drucker, Peter, 219
DrugAbacus, 132–3
drugs, *see* medication
Dubos, René, 37

eculizumab (drug), 23
Ehrenreich, Barbara, 205
Emanuel, Rahm, 220
end-of-life care, 206–16, 256–7
EpiPens, 96
EQRx (Biotechnology company), 250
European Cancer Medicines Agency, 215
Evaluate Pharma, 107
Express Scripts, 133

'Fair Society, Healthy Lives' (Marmot), 150–52
fever hospitals, 48
Finland, 75
Food and Drug Administration (FDA), 23, 103, 129
Forbes magazine, 106–7
France, 70, 128
Franklin, Benjamin, 54
Frome, Somerset, 199, 244–5
Future Hospital Commission, 57

Gandhi, Mahatma, 76
Garrett, Laurie, 136
Gawande, Atul, 86–7, 209, 212, 246
General Medical Council (GMC), 16
genomics, 23, 217, 232–6
  genetic testing, 234–5
Genomics Plc, 235
George V, king of the United Kingdom, 192

INDEX

Germany, 70–71, 128
  Health Insurance Act (1883), 70
Ghebreyesus, Tedros Adhanom, 36, 69
Gilead Sciences (pharmaceutical company), 130–31
Giuliani, Rudy, 171–2
Glasziou, Paul, 171
Global Justice Now, 99
'Good Medical Practice'(GMC), 16
Gove, Michael, 139
GPs, *see* doctors
GRAIL study, 234
Guardian, 19, 95, 116

Hancock, Matt, 9, 198, 225, 234–5
Harvoni (drug), 131
health check-ups, 197
Health Connections Mendip, 199
Health Education England, 57
Health Foundation, 135
health insurance, 25–6, 66, 112–14, 118
Health Japan 21 initiative, 196
Health Services Journal, 182
healthcare, 22–3
  aspirations, 258–60
  boundaries of, 250–52
  budgets, 135–6, 239
  cost-effectiveness, 129–33, 247–9
  costs, 25–37, 42–3, 58–63, 64–7, 85–6
  expectations, 82–3
  expenditure (worldwide), 79–82
  expenses, 67
  politics and, 12, 18–19, 25, 33, 35, 58, 61, 69–70, 145, 171, 239–41, 250
  'rationing', 115–19, 252
healthcare administrators, 17–18
healthy lifestyle, 196–7
heart disease, *see* cardiovascular disease
hepatitis C, 130–31

Herceptin (drug), 66
high blood pressure, 53, 158–60, 175
hip replacements, 65–7
Hippocrates, 213
HIV/AIDS, 93–4
hospices, 207–8
hospitals, 49, 208, 214, 249
  fever hospitals, 48
  Nightingale hospitals, 9–10, 13
'How American Medicine Is Destroying Itself' (Callahan & Nuland), 246
Huffington Post, 129
Humana (US health insurance company), 26
Hunt, Jeremy, 90
Hurricane Katrina (2005), 77
Huxley, Aldous, 163

Iceland, 75
immunization, *see* vaccination
Improving Access to Psychological Therapies, 182
India, 36
Indonesia, 36
infant mortality, 41
influenza, 48
Institute for Clinical and Economic Review (ICER), 130–31, 133
Institute for Fiscal Studies, 5
Institute for Healthcare Improvement, 22
Institute for Work and Health, Canada, 141–2
Institute of Health and Welfare, Australia, 152–3
International Federation of Health Plans, 65
internet, 241
'inverse care law', 51, 67
Ireland, 251
Italy, 11, 238–9, 253

INDEX

JAMA Internal Medicine, 99
Japan, 70, 75, 194, 196–7
Jenner Institute, Oxford, 106
Jenner, Edward, 134
Johnson, Boris, 2, 5, 20, 244
Johnson, Wilko, 117
Journal of Oncology, 108
Journal of the American Medical Association, 101, 253

Kenber, Billy, 100
Kent, Jennifer, 32
King's Fund (UK), 174, 194, 243, 254
Kingston, Helen, 244
Kirkwood, Tom, 54

Lancet, The, 29, 33, 53
'Leadership and Management for All Doctors' (GMC), 16
Lehman, Richard, 214
'Levelling Up Health' report, 11
Levitin, Daniel, 191, 193
levothyroxine sodium, 110
Lieberman, Daniel, 193
life expectancy, 3, 13, 38–42, 54–5, 85, 192–6, 236
  Covid-19 and, 39–41
  deprivation and, 195
  diminishing returns, 193
  education and, 195
  geographical variation, 194
  'healthy life expectancy', 194–8
  healthy lifestyle, 196–7
Lincoln, Abraham, 191
litigation, 89–90
Lloyd George, David, 71
lobbying, 89, 130, 132
loneliness, 19–20, 199–203, 244
low-value care, 26–7
LSE–Lancet Commission, 5, 13
lupus erythematosus, 29
Luxturna (drug), 23

Mackenzie, James, 48, 50
Macmillan Cancer Relief, 15
Marie Curie charity, 206
Marmot, Michael, 40, 150–52, 195
Marshall, Martin, 226, 258
Matsoso, Malebona Precious, 104
McBain, Sophie, 202–3
McCain, John, 210
Mead, Rebecca, 202
measles, 138
medical equipment, cost of, 64–5, 84
Medical Journal of Australia, 171
medical practices, 43–6
medical procedures
  cost of, 65–7
  overuse of, 87–9, 254
medication, 19–20, 74–5
  affordability, 112–15
  cost of drugs, 23–4, 30, 66, 91–111, 250
  cost-effectiveness, 119–33, 246–7
  overprescribing, 91–3
  patents, 102–3
  'rationing', 115–18
  see also pharmaceutical industry
Memorial Sloan Kettering Cancer Center, 132
Mencken, H. L., 155
mental health, 24, 82–3, 181–9
  depression, 161–2, 186–8
  funding, 188–9
  suicide, 83, 161–2, 183
  young people and, 182
'mental health first aid', 188
Mental Health Foundation, 183
Mirage of Health (Dubos), *37*
misdiagnosis, 173–5, 254–5
MMR vaccine, 140
Moderna (biotech firm), 106–7
Montori, Victor, 257–8
Moran, Lord, *see* Wilson, Charles, 1st Baron Moran

INDEX

motorcycle accidents, 137–8
Moynihan, Ray, 177
MRI scanners, 64–6
Mulley, Al, 174, 254–5
multimorbidity, 55–7, 85, 241
multiple sclerosis, 29
Murthy, Vivek, 200
Mylan (pharmaceutical company), 96

Nakajima, Hiroshi, 194
National Academy for Social Prescribing, 201
National Center for Health Care Technology (US), 129
National Health Service (NHS), 12–13, 72–5, 165–6, 242–3, 250–51
  cost of drugs, 23–4, 30–31, 102, 246
  cost of drugs, 91–2, 111, 119–20
  cost-effectiveness, 248–9
  costs, 58–9, 73–4
  decision-making, 166–7
  establishment of, 28, 38, 71–4
  funding, 2–7, 11, 24–5, 28, 70–71
  litigation, 89–90
  NHS Long Term Plan, 148
  NHS Resolution, 90
  'one-stop shops', 249
  prescription charges, 74
  primary care and, 148
  staff, 10, 85–6, 149, 259
  underfunding, 4–5, 25
  see also doctors; National Institute for Health and Care Excellence (NICE)
National Institute for Health and Care Excellence (NICE), 19, 87, 119–20, 122–8, 133, 167, 215, 246, 249–51
National Insurance Act (1911), 71–2
National Palliative and End of Life Care Partnership, 207
National Programme for IT, 228–9

Natural Causes: Life, Death and the Illusion of Control (Ehrenreich), 205
Nature Reviews Clinical Oncology, 109
Nature Reviews Neuroscience, 203
New England Journal of Medicine, 233
New Statesman, 202
New York Times, 29, 79, 102, 131, 132, 133
New Yorker, 86, 202
New Zealand, 75, 129
Nicholson, David, 10
Nightingale hospitals, 9–10, 13
Northern Echo, 119
Norway, 59, 62, 75
Novartis (pharmaceutical company), 23, 111
Nuland, Sherwin B., 246
'number needed to treat' (NNT), 160–61
nursing homes, 213

obesity, 142, 150, 164
Office of Technology Assessment (US), 129
Oliver, David, 211
omeprazole, 110
Organization for Economic Cooperation and Development (OECD), 197
'orphan drugs', 102–3
Osborne, George, 25
over-definition, 175–9
overdetection, 173–5, 254–5
overdiagnosis, *see* diagnosis
overmedicalization, 19–20, 161
overtreatment, 155–79
oxytocin (hormone), 231

Palin, Sarah, 118
palliative care, 209–16, 256–7
pandemics, 21; *see also* Covid-19
'parity of esteem', 183–5

INDEX

paroxysmal nocturnal haemoglobinuria, 23
patents, 102–3, 250
patient choice, 31–2, 125–6, 173–5, 204–5, 254–5
patient-centred care, 214–15
'Patients' Preferences Matter' (Mulley), 254
Payer, Lynn, 175–6
peptic ulcers, 43–4, 46
Personalised Care Institute, 255
personalized medicine, 23–4, 56–7, 236
Petty, Duncan, 92
Pfizer (pharmaceutical company), 94–5, 107
Pharmaceutical Benefits Advisory Committee, Australia, 128
pharmaceutical industry, 93–101, 233–4, 250
 anti-cancer drugs, 107–9
 Covid-19 and, 106–7
 discounts, 105
 'disease mongering', 175–7
 government funding, 99–100
 international market, 103–4
 lobbying power, 130, 132
 marketing, 101–2
 patents, 102–3
 profits, 105–6
 research and development, 97–100, 102, 104
 see also medication
Pharmaceutical Management Agency, New Zealand, 129
Philippines, 36
PLOS Medicine, 204
pneumonia, 3, 46, 48
Portugal, 70
Praluent (drug), 133
prediabetes, 162–3
'preference misdiagnosis', 173–5, 254–5

pregnenolone (hormone), 199
prescription drugs, *see* medication
preventative healthcare, 18, 22–3, 134–54
 decision-making, 165–8
 guidelines, 164–5
 primary prevention, 136–7
 secondary and tertiary prevention, 140–43
 vaccination, 13, 18, 134, 138–9
 see also primary care
primary care, 146–50
Primary Health Care Performance Initiative, 146–7
Prospect magazine, 170
public health, *see* healthcare

quality-adjusted life year (QALY), 122–5, 128, 133
Quality and Outcomes Framework (QOF), 221
quality of life, 121–4

Read, Ian, 94–5
research and development (R&D), 79, 97–100
respiratory disease, 46
rheumatoid arthritis, 187
Rivett, Geoffrey, 72
robotics, 223, 230–32
Royal College of Physicians, 57
Russia, 75

Salama, Peter, 147
Scobie, Sarah, 216
Scotland, 56
Scott Morton, Fiona, 131
screening, 155–8, 168–9, 172–3
self-care, 242–3
Shakespeare, William, 219
Shrank, William, 26

INDEX

Sick Money (Kember), 100
smallpox vaccine, 48, 135
'Smart Life Project', 196–7
Smith, Richard, 210
smoking, 53, 135, 142, 150
Snow, John, 135
social care, 13, 256–7
social inequality, 11–12, 24, 39–41, 51–2, 56–7, 150–53
   life expectancy and, 39–42, 151, 195–6
'social isolation syndrome', 19
'social prescribing', 201–2
Soriot, Pascal, 95–6
South Africa, 36
South Korea, 75, 128, 174
Sovaldi (drug), 130–31
Spain, 12, 70
specialisation, 48–9, 57–8, 241
Spiegelhalter, David, 170
spinal muscular atrophy, 23, 111
Starfield, Barbara, 147
statins, 110, 166–7
Stevens, Simon, 12–13
Stevenson, Robert Louis, 192
Stokes-Lampard, Helen, 176, 201
strokes, *see* cardiovascular disease
suicide, 83, 161–2, 183
Sunak, Rishi, 2
Sunday Times, The, 95
Suprun, Ulana, 33
Sweden, 12, 70, 75, 75
Swiss Re Institute, 235

Taiwan, 75
technological development, 217–29
Thailand, 75, 128
Times, The, 49, 90, 95, 98, 106, 172, 256
tisagenlecleucel (drug), 109, 237
touch, 231
Trump, Donald, 2, 139
tuberculosis, 46, 48
Tudor Hart, Julian, 51–2
Tufts Center for the Study of Drug Development, 98–9
Tutu, Desmond, 142

'Uncertainty and the Welfare Economics of Medical Care' (Arrow), 31–2
United Nations, 68–9, 103–4, 191
   Sustainable Development Goals, 69
United States, 12, 22–3, 140, 160
   cardiovascular disease, 186
   coronary heart disease and, 51
   cost of drugs, 91–2, 109, 111
   cost-effectiveness analysis, 129–33, 247–9
   diabetes, 163
   end-of-life care, 209
   health insurance, 25–6, 66, 113
   healthcare costs, 28–30, 58–9, 66, 86–7, 118–19
   healthcare funding, 77–9
   healthcare in, 25–6, 71, 77–81
   healthcare inequality, 78–81, 152
   life expectancy in, 39, 78, 192
   litigation, 90
   Medicare programme, 86–7, 129, 215
   mental health, 162, 181
   motorcycle accidents, 137–8
   Preventive Services Task Force, 172
   primary care and, 149–50
   preventative medicine, 171–3
   suicide, 161, 183
   see also medication; pharmaceutical industry
'universal health coverage' (UHC), 68–70, 75–6
universal healthcare systems, 15–16

INDEX

vaccination, 13, 18, 31, 134, 138–9
  anti-vax campaign, 138–9
'value-based insurance design', 133
virtual consultations, 60–61

Wakefield, Andrew, 140
Wall Street Journal, 111
Wanless, Derek, 242–3
Warneford Hospital, Leamington Spa, 43
Watt, Graham, 52
'Whitehall II' (Marmot), 195–6
Why We Revolt (Montori), 257

Wilson, Charles, 1st Baron Moran, 49
World Health Assembly, Geneva, 144
World Health Organization (WHO), 11, 60, 67–70, 121, 128, 146–7, 157–8, 181–2, 187, 223
World Mental Health survey (WHO), 181–2
World Psychiatry, 181
World War II (1939–45), 72, 74–5

Zaltrap (drug), 232
Zolgensma (drug), 23, 111

A Note About the Author

Sir David Haslam is former chair of NICE, a former president of the Royal College of GPs and a former president of the British Medical Association. He practised as a General Practitioner in Cambridgeshire for over 35 years, has written over 2000 articles and papers for the medical and lay press and has been invited to speak at conferences in 33 different countries. In 2014 he was named by *Debretts* and the *Sunday Times* as one of the 500 most influential and inspirational people in the United Kingdom.